Children's Neuromuscular Disorders

Michael Benson • John Fixsen • Malcolm Macnicol
Klaus Parsch
Editors

Children's Neuromuscular Disorders

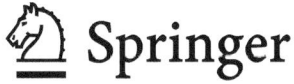

Editors

Michael Benson
Ridgway
Harberton Mead
OX3 ODB Oxford
United Kingdom
michael.benson@doctors.org.uk

John Fixsen
West Barn
Clamok Farm Barns
Wier Quay
PL20 7BU Bere Alston
United Kingdom
jafixsen@btinternet.com

Malcolm Macnicol
Red House
Gillsland Road 1
EH10 5DE Edinburgh
United Kingdom
mmacnicol@aol.com

Klaus Parsch
Weinbergweg 68
70569 Stuttgart Baden-
Württemberg
Germany
kparsch@t-online.de

ISBN 978-0-85729-551-4   e-ISBN 978-0-85729-552-1
DOI 10.1007/978-0-85729-552-1
Springer London Dordrecht Heidelberg New York

British Library Cataloguing in Publication Data
A catalogue record for this book is available from the British Library

Library of Congress Control Number: 2011929878

Cover design: eStudio Calamar S.L.

Printed on acid-free paper

Springer is part of Springer Science+Business Media (www.springer.com)

Foreword

Confirming the British genetic trait for writing and publishing (as well as acting), two English (Oxford and London) and a Scottish orthopaedic surgeon (Edinburgh) have produced a third edition of their comprehensive text, joined, as in the second edition by an editor from Germany, recognizing its part in the European community. The 62 physician contributors are drawn from pink-colored countries in our childhood geography books—the old British Empire from Australia to Zambia and two from the former colony, the USA.

The original purpose of the book was to give residents or registrars an easily accessible and concise description of diseases and conditions encountered in the practice of paediatric orthopaedic surgery and to prepare for their examinations. But the practicing orthopaedic surgeon will find an update of current practice that can be read for clarity and constraint—enough but not too much. A foreword might be a preview of things to come, but a "back word" of what was thought to be the final say on the subject is needed for a perspective in progress.

A "back word" look reveals the tremendous progress in medical diagnosis and treatment of which paediatric orthopaedics and fracture care is a component. Clubfoot treatment based on the dictums of Hiram Kite has had a revolutionary change by Ponseti. The chapter by Eastwood has the details on cast application and orthotics follow-up to obtain the 95% correction without the extensive surgery many of us thought was needed.

Paediatric fracture care has also changed from traction for fractures of the femoral shaft in the ages of 5–15 years to intramedullary fixation with elastic stable nails originated in Nancy and Metz, France—"Nancy nails." Klaus Parsch's chapter tells us that it is their preferred method of treatment in Stuttgart, Germany.

Robert Dickson's lucid writing on idiopathic scoliosis as primarily a rotation of the lordotic thoracic spine again bears study to deepen the understanding that it is a three-dimensional deformity. As in the past editions, a coat hanger helps to appreciate the distortion of curvatures in a one-dimensional radiograph. Those orthopaedists who need courage to resist pressure to encase children in casts or braces or orthoses will be heartened to know that none of these conservative measures have shown any effect in prevention or curve progression. What to do instead of "treatment"? Read on.

This is not a book to learn the details of surgical technique–other texts and only experience can do that. Even though a seasoned orthopaedic surgeon does not need this knowledge to pass an examination, he or she is expected to know something about the subject. Once identified as an orthopaedic surgeon, your opinion is often sought at social events usually standing with a drink in hand. And commonly it is advice sought by your married children about a grandchild's musculoskeletal problem. Can you answer sensibly? If, "I'll get back to you later" is your response, a quick perusal of the contents of this volume should help maintain your professional standing and as is now the fashion of school teachers, your "self-esteem." And you won't have to log on to the Internet.

Eugene E Bleck

Preface

The newborn child's immature nervous system makes early diagnosis of some neurological disorders difficult: it is often only the passage of time which clarifies the severity and pattern. Careful analysis of motor skills, vision, hearing and speech allows us to assess milestones. Progress from head control to sitting, standing and the maturation of gait should be orderly. Informed examination and the chapter on gait analysis highlight this development. Chapters in this section describe neural tube defects, the recognition and management of cerebral palsy and, lest we forget, poliomyelitis. The section is completed by considering the muscular dystrophies and arthrogryposis.

Michael KD Benson, Oxford, UK   John A Fixsen, London, UK
Malcolm F Macnicol, Edinburgh, UK   Klaus Parsch, Stuttgart, Germany

June, 2011

Contents

Contributors

Eugene E. Bleck Department of Orthopaedic Surgery, Stanford University School of Medicine, Stanford, CA, USA

Reinald G. Brunner Department of Neuro-Orthopaedics, University Children's Hospital Basel, Basel, Switzerland

Wang Chow Department of Orthopaedics and Traumatology, Hong Kong, China

John A. Fixsen Orthopaedic Department, Great Ormond Street Hospital for Sick Children, London, UK

H. Kerr Graham Department of Orthopaedics, The Royal Children's Hospital, Parkville, Victoria, Australia

Göran Hansson Department of Pediatric Surgery, The Queen Silvia Children's Hospital, Goteborg, Sweden

F. Stig Jacobsen Orthopaedics Department, Marshfield Clinic, Marshfield, WI, USA

Chi Yan John Leong The Open University of Hong Kong, Hong Kong, China

Yun Hoi Li Departments of Orthopaedics and Traumatology, Hong Kong Pediatric Orthopaedics Centre, Hong Kong, China

Robert A. Minns Department of Child Life and Health, University of Edinburgh, Edinburgh, UK; Royal Hospital for Sick Children, Edinburgh, UK

Klaus Parsch Orthopaedic Department, Pediatric Centre Olgahospital, Stuttgart, Germany

James E. Robb Department of Orthopaedic Surgery, Edinburgh, UK; Royal Hospital for Sick Children, Edinburgh, UK; University of Edinburgh; University of St. Andrews; Edinburgh, UK

Tim N. Theologis Nuffield Orthopaedic Centre, Oxford, UK

Chapter 1

Gait Analysis

Tim N. Theologis

Normal Gait

Definitions

The term *gait* describes the characteristics of body motion during walking or running. The study of bipedal gait in humans is called *gait analysis* and refers to the objective and systematic study of human locomotion, including both visual observation and measurement using instrumentation.

Normal gait is a complex activity that relies on control by the central nervous system and the integrity of the spinal cord, peripheral nerves, and the musculoskeletal system. Its purpose is to propel the body forward while maintaining an upright posture and conserving energy. The neurological control of gait is based on an automated central nervous system mechanism, which may be modified by visual, sensory (including somatosensory), and acoustic stimuli while it remains under voluntary control.

From the biomechanical viewpoint, the prerequisites of normal gait include stability of the weight-bearing limb, appropriate pre-positioning of the limb for initial contact, adequate clearance of the non-weight-bearing limb, efficient step length, and energy conservation [1]. In order to achieve these, normal neurological control and an intact musculoskeletal system are necessary.

The description of gait is based on the definition of its unit, the *gait cycle*. The gait cycle is the period of time between the initial contact of one foot with the ground and its next contact with the ground. The timing of events occurring during a gait cycle is usually described as a percentage of this cycle, considering the initial contact as 0% and the second contact of the same foot as 100%. The gait cycle is divided into *stance phase* when the limb under consideration is in contact with the ground and *swing phase* when the limb is off the ground

and moving forward. Stance occupies approximately 60% of the cycle and swing the remaining 40%.

Another important subdivision of the gait cycle is into single and double limb support time. At initial contact both feet are on the ground, the first double support phase. At about 10% through the cycle the contralateral limb lifts off the ground. At this point double support time finishes and single support time commences. Fifty percent through the cycle, the contralateral limb contacts the ground again, which marks the beginning of the second double support time of the cycle; this finishes at the end of stance phase of the first limb 60% through the cycle. Therefore, there are two periods of double limb support time at the beginning and the end of the stance phase, each lasting 10% of the cycle.

Walking speed, usually expressed in meters per second, depends on cadence (steps per minute) and stride length (the sum of left and right step lengths). Stride time and step time are often measured in the temporal and spatial assessment of gait.

Description of Normal Gait

Systematic description of gait should always consider all three anatomical planes: sagittal, coronal, and transverse. Consideration should also be given to all moving body segments, including the head, upper limbs, trunk, pelvis, and lower limbs (see Fig. 1.1). A detailed description of motion in the lower limb segments and joints will follow later in this section.

Human gait characteristics depend on age, anatomical/structural characteristics, and walking speed. Each individual has a preferred or self-selected speed, which is optimal for energy conservation. Deviations from this optimal speed alter gait characteristics. Despite these individual variations, human gait characteristics are largely universal and the inter- and intra-subject variations are relatively small. When considering pathological gait, however, the variability of normal gait patterns should be taken into account. Some perceived

T.N. Theologis (✉)
Nuffield Orthopaedic Centre, Oxford, UK

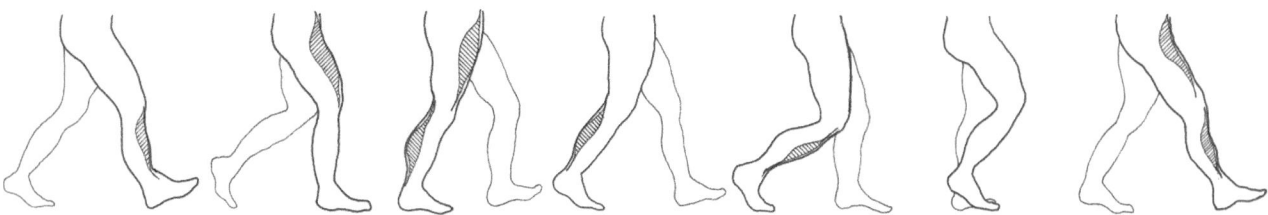

Fig. 1.1 The gait cycle subdivided into stance including initial contact, loading response, mid-stance, and late stance; and swing including initial, mid, and terminal swing. The predominant muscle activation during each phase is also shown

gait abnormalities may be normal variants or compensations for other underlying problems.

The gait cycle begins with the initial contact of the heel with the ground, often described as *heelstrike*. To achieve heel contact the foot is in neutral plantar/dorsiflexion and this requires activation of the dorsiflexors. The knee is slightly flexed at 5–10° and the hip is flexed at 30°. Following initial contact, the foot plantarflexes in relation to the tibia to allow forefoot ground contact. This is known as the *first ankle rocker* and is controlled by eccentric contraction of the dorsiflexors (see Fig. 1.2). In this early part of stance, knee flexion increases to 15–20° to allow smooth acceptance of body weight onto the weight-bearing limb. This increase in flexion is known as the *loading response* and is controlled by eccentric quadriceps activity. It coincides with the first double support time and is also characterized by progressive extension of the hip, driven by the gluteal muscles and the hamstrings. Mid-stance commences at the point of the opposite foot toe-off. During mid-stance the knee and hip progressively extend fully. At the hip, extension occurs passively through inertia. Some quadriceps activity is necessary at the knee to control the speed of flexion. While the weight-bearing foot remains in contact with the ground, the tibia progresses forward over it and the whole body is propelled forward. This is described as the *second ankle rocker* and is controlled by an eccentric contraction of the triceps surae.

In late stance, the foot plantarflexes on the tibia as the concentric contraction of the triceps surae propels the body forward. This phase is known as push-off or the *third ankle rocker*. The knee begins to flex at this stage in order to reach the flexion required in swing phase. The hip remains extended until the end of stance.

During initial swing the ankle dorsiflexes rapidly toward neutral through concentric contraction of the dorsiflexors. At the same time the knee and hip flex rapidly to allow clearance of the foot from the ground. Proximally, the iliopsoas actively flexes the hip. Knee flexion is a passive pendulum effect of the hip flexion. The knee reaches over 60° of flexion within the initial third of swing. Any pathology preventing this flexion results in foot clearance problems (e.g., spasticity of the rectus femoris muscle).

In mid-swing, the foot passes the opposite weight-bearing side and actively dorsiflexes further. The knee extends while the hip remains flexed. There is little muscle activity at hip and knee during this stage.

In terminal swing, the foot lowers toward the ground and dorsiflexion reduces. This is controlled by the dorsiflexors. At the knee, concentric activity of the quadriceps and eccentric activity of the hamstrings drive the knee toward extension. The hip remains flexed at 30°.

In the coronal plane there is a limited range of pelvic motion. The weight-bearing side is higher than the opposite one and the hip on the swing side is slightly abducted. In the transverse plane there is also a small range of pelvic rotation, which remains normally within 5–10° and aids forward propulsion. The hips rotate slightly around the neutral position and maximum internal rotation occurs in terminal stance. Foot progression (the angle between the axis of the

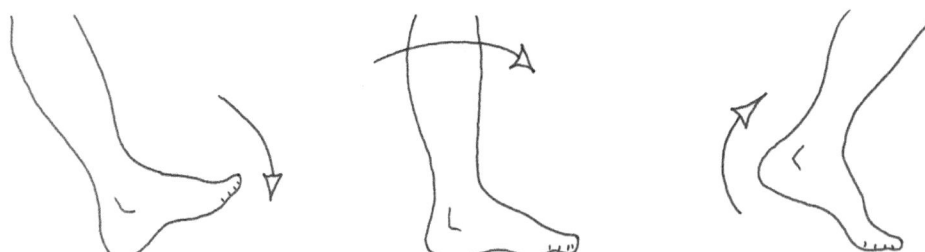

Fig. 1.2 The three ankle rockers. During the first rocker, the heel contacts the ground and the foot plantarflexes to allow the sole and forefoot to reach the ground. During the second rocker, the foot remains in contact with the ground, while the tibia progresses forward over it, producing dorsiflexion at ankle level. During the third rocker, the foot plantarflexes again to lift the heel off the ground and push forward

foot and the line of gait progression) is normally between 0° and 30° external rotation.

The upper body moves forward during walking but its speed is variable, accelerating during double support and decelerating during single support. The trunk also moves up and down twice during the gait cycle. The highest points coincide with mid-stance and mid-swing. In the coronal plane there is lateral leaning of the trunk toward the weight-bearing limb. In the transverse plane, the shoulders and trunk rotate toward the opposite direction in relation to the pelvis. The arms swing out of phase with the lower limbs. The leg swings forward simultaneously with the arm and shoulder of the opposite side.

The *ground reaction force* is important as it influences the stability of gait in general and the lower limb joints in particular. The fore-aft or antero-posterior component of the force vector is directed posteriorly in early and mid-stance, as a braking mechanism tending to decelerate the forward movement of the body. During transition from mid- to late stance the direction of the ground reaction force becomes anterior to contribute toward the forward acceleration of the body (see Fig. 1.3). The lateral component of the ground reaction force

is relatively small and the direction of acceleration is toward the non-weight-bearing limb during most of stance.

The acceleration and deceleration of body speed coincide with energy conversion between potential and kinetic. During the first double support time, the body is at its lowest position and at its highest speed. Following this, kinetic energy is converted to potential energy and the body reaches its highest position and slowest speed during single support. Later in stance, the body lowers again and its speed increases. The rotation of the shoulders and pelvis in opposite directions is another example of an exchange between kinetic and potential energy.

Development of Gait

Gait Maturation

Most infants achieve independent bipedal walking at 12–18 months. Infant gait, characterized by its broad base of support, persists for 2–3 years. The arms are usually held up and out for balance and reciprocal swinging is not achieved until the age of 4–5 years. Infants make initial contact with the foot flat on the ground and the hip externally rotated while there is no knee flexion for loading response. Heel strike, normal hip rotation, and loading response are achieved around the age of 2 years. Although most infants walk with external hip rotation, some with persistent foetal alignment have an in-toe gait. Increased femoral anteversion, internal tibial torsion, metatarsus adductus, or a combination of these rotational variations may lead to internal foot progression.

Stride length depends on leg length and is, therefore, height and age dependent. Infants compensate for their reduced stride length by increasing their cadence. By the age of 7–8 years, their speed and cadence, normalized for height, are similar to that of an adult. In absolute terms, children achieve normal adult walking speed around the age of 12–15 years. It should be noted here that speed affects gait parameters, including kinematics and kinetics. Therefore, when assessing gait parameters, walking speed as well as the subject's anthropometric parameters (height or leg length) should be taken into account [2].

Electromyographic studies have shown that infants activate their lower limb muscles for longer periods during the walking cycle but reach adult patterns by the age of 2 years [3].

Variations of Gait

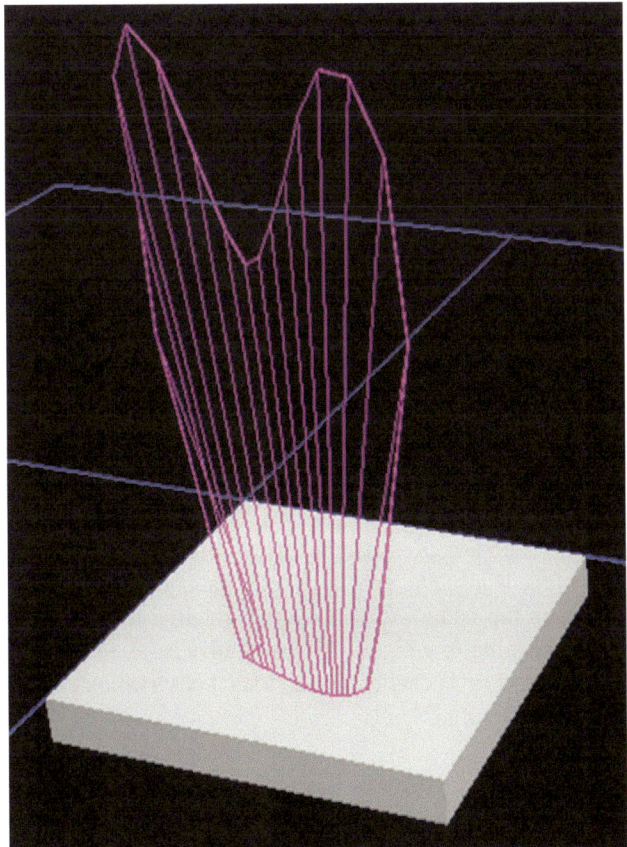

Fig. 1.3 The butterfly-shaped diagram of the ground reaction force throughout stance

Most children achieve independent ambulation by the age of 18 months. Children who are late in achieving their motor milestones may achieve independent walking later. After 18 months children who are not walking require assessment to rule out an underlying neurological or orthopaedic condition that could be responsible for the delay.

It is not uncommon for toddlers to walk weight bearing on the forefoot only when they start to walk. Such "toe-walking" is common up to the age of 2 years but prolonged or acquired toe-walking should be investigated for an underlying neurological condition or the plantarflexor tightness often seen in idiopathic toe-walking.

Children may use a variety of compensatory mechanisms for leg length discrepancy. Small discrepancies are compensated in the coronal plane by tilting the pelvis down on the short side. This is accompanied by hip adduction on the higher side of the pelvis and hip abduction on the shorter side. A compensatory postural scoliosis may develop. In larger discrepancies, increased plantarflexion on the short side or *vaulting* may be observed. Increased flexion of the hip and knee and dorsiflexion of the foot on the long side are additional compensatory mechanisms for leg length inequality. In order to aid clearance of the longer limb in swing phase, increased hip and knee flexion or hip circumduction in swing may be employed. When these variations of gait are seen, careful clinical assessment is needed to identify the primary problem. If there is no true leg length discrepancy, structural spinal deformity, joint, or muscle contracture may be responsible. It should also be noted that late-diagnosed hip dysplasia often presents as gait asymmetry and leg length inequality.

Gait asymmetry due to lower limb pain is associated with a variety of musculoskeletal conditions, including trauma. This type of gait is often described as antalgic. Its main characteristic is the short stance phase on the affected side. Other secondary characteristics depend on the pain site and the nature of the underlying condition.

Compensations around the pelvis are often observed in response to hip pathology. The Trendelenburg gait is characterized by hip adduction on the affected weight-bearing side and coronal plane pelvic obliquity, with the affected side being higher than the opposite side. The trunk leans toward the weight-bearing side. This type of gait is caused by hip instability and/or weakness or insufficiency of the hip abductors. In Duchenne gait, the pelvis rotates toward the affected weight-bearing hip in the coronal plane. The hip is therefore abducted during weight bearing. The trunk leans toward the affected weight-bearing side.

neurological conditions can affect it. Important information that may influence diagnosis and treatment is revealed by observation and analysis of gait. This information should be evaluated together with the patient's history, clinical examination, and other diagnostic investigations.

The particular parameters of walking that need analysis and the complexity of the necessary assessment should be determined on an individual patient basis. Instrumented three-dimensional gait analysis using sophisticated equipment is well established for patients with cerebral palsy. Gait analysis for less difficult conditions, such as an isolated leg length discrepancy or drop foot, requires less sophisticated techniques.

An understanding of the capabilities and limitations of the various techniques will avoid over- or under-interpretation of results. Gait analysis is also an important measure of the outcome of treatment. When the aim of treatment is to improve walking, it is essential that gait is objectively evaluated before and after treatment.

Observational Analysis

Systematic observation of gait should form part of the orthopaedic clinical examination. The three anatomical planes should be considered and observation should involve all the mobile segments of the body. The patient's gait should be compared with normal patterns. Deviations of gait that compromise the prerequisites of gait should be given particular attention. Slow-motion video or digital imaging can assist with the detailed assessment of walking. Systematic observation can be enhanced by using validated scores, such as the Edinburgh visual gait score [4].

A significant limitation of observational gait analysis is the difficulty in discriminating between movements that occur in more than one of the three anatomical planes. The degree of knee flexion in the sagittal plane, for example, may be significantly underestimated if the hip is internally rotated at the time of observation. Another typical example of this limitation of visual gait analysis relates to the scissoring of the legs at hip level in diplegic patients: discrimination between hip adduction and internal rotation in this context is challenging (see Fig. 1.4). Quantitative assessment of gait deviations is also challenging by visual observation alone.

Analysis of Gait

Gait assessment is an integral part of the clinical evaluation of the patient. A multitude of musculoskeletal and

Kinematics

The study of kinematics, as part of gait analysis, describes the motion of body segments. It includes their position and

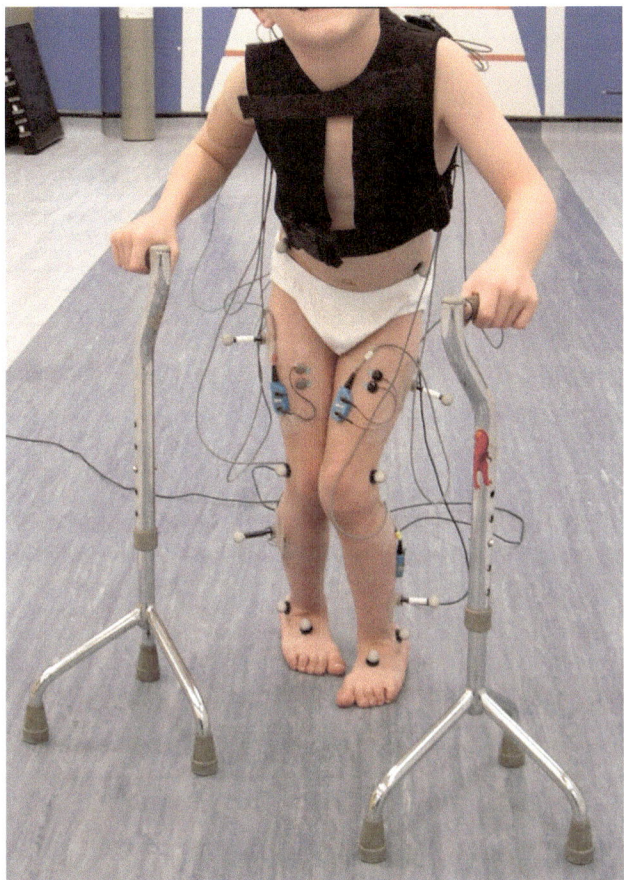

Fig. 1.4 Limitations of observational gait analysis. Discriminating between hip adduction and internal rotation in this patient would be challenging. Quantifying the degree of adduction and/or internal rotation would not be possible through simple observation

orientation, the angles of the joints, and the corresponding linear and angular velocities and accelerations.

Typically, three-dimensional kinematic analysis involves optico-electronic cameras tracking markers placed on anatomical landmarks of the body. The information on the position of the markers is digitized through an appropriate interface. A computerized biomechanical model of the musculoskeletal system is then used to convert the information on the position and movement of the markers to a description of body movements. The output usually involves the graphic representation of individual joint movements during the gait cycle (see Fig. 1.5). Comparison of those graphs with a normal database offers a quantification of the gait deviations observed in the individual patient. State-of-the-art equipment can acquire images at 100 Hz with accuracy of under 1 mm.

Instrumented kinematic analysis can provide accurate, detailed, and quantifiable information on the motion of body segments in the three anatomical planes. It is an objective assessment method which offers invaluable information for managing patients and in evaluating the outcome of treatment. Its main limitation is that it relies on a sophisticated and expensive laboratory setup, which assesses walking on level ground and does not necessarily reproduce real-life conditions. Furthermore, interpretation of gait data is complex and requires specific training.

Kinematic data can also be expressed in terms of muscle length variation (as opposed to angular joint changes). This offers potentially useful information, particularly in neuromuscular conditions. The current biomechanical muscle models, however, are susceptible to error, particularly when anatomical variations and deformities coexist.

Electrogoniometers can be attached to the limbs to measure the dynamic range of joint motion during gait. They are portable but less precise than conventional kinematic equipment. Accelerometers and gyroscopes have also been introduced: they measure, respectively, the acceleration and orientation of body segments. While they can record data for long periods of time and can be used during activities of daily living, they lack precision by comparison with conventional gait analysis.

Kinetics

The information obtained from kinematic analysis can be combined with information obtained from a force platform set into the floor, which measures the ground reaction force of a single step. This combination of data helps to calculate the *inverse dynamics*, a close estimate of the forces and moments acting on individual segments and joints, together with the power generation or absorption in these areas. These data help our understanding of gait deviations and the discrimination between true gait problems and compensations. The output is similar to the kinematic data: Individual joint kinetic variations are shown graphically against time during the gait cycle.

Dynamic Electromyography

Dynamic electromyography (EMG) records the electrical signals from muscles during walking. Multiple muscles can be recorded simultaneously and the signals compared with published or lab-based data of normal phasic activity. Muscles produce EMG signals with any type of contraction, whether concentric, isometric, or eccentric. Furthermore, the intensity of the EMG signal is not indicative of the force generated by the muscle.

For the purposes of gait analysis, most EMGs are obtained using surface electrodes attached to the skin. Fine wires inserted through a needle can be used for deep muscles, such as the tibialis posterior and gluteus medius. In combination with kinematic and kinetic data, EMGs can contribute toward the understanding of gait deviations.

Fig. 1.5 Example of normal kinematic graphs. The left column of graphs represents the sagittal plane, the middle one the coronal, and the right one the transverse. Lower limb joints and segments as shown from proximal (*top*) to distal (*bottom*). The *x*-axis of each graph represents the percentage of the gait cycle. The *y*-axis represents the joint angle. Each curve, therefore, shows the variation of the relevant joint angle during the gait cycle. Right and left leg angles are superimposed in each graph. The vertical line in each graph represents the separation between stance and swing phase at approximately 60% of the gait cycle

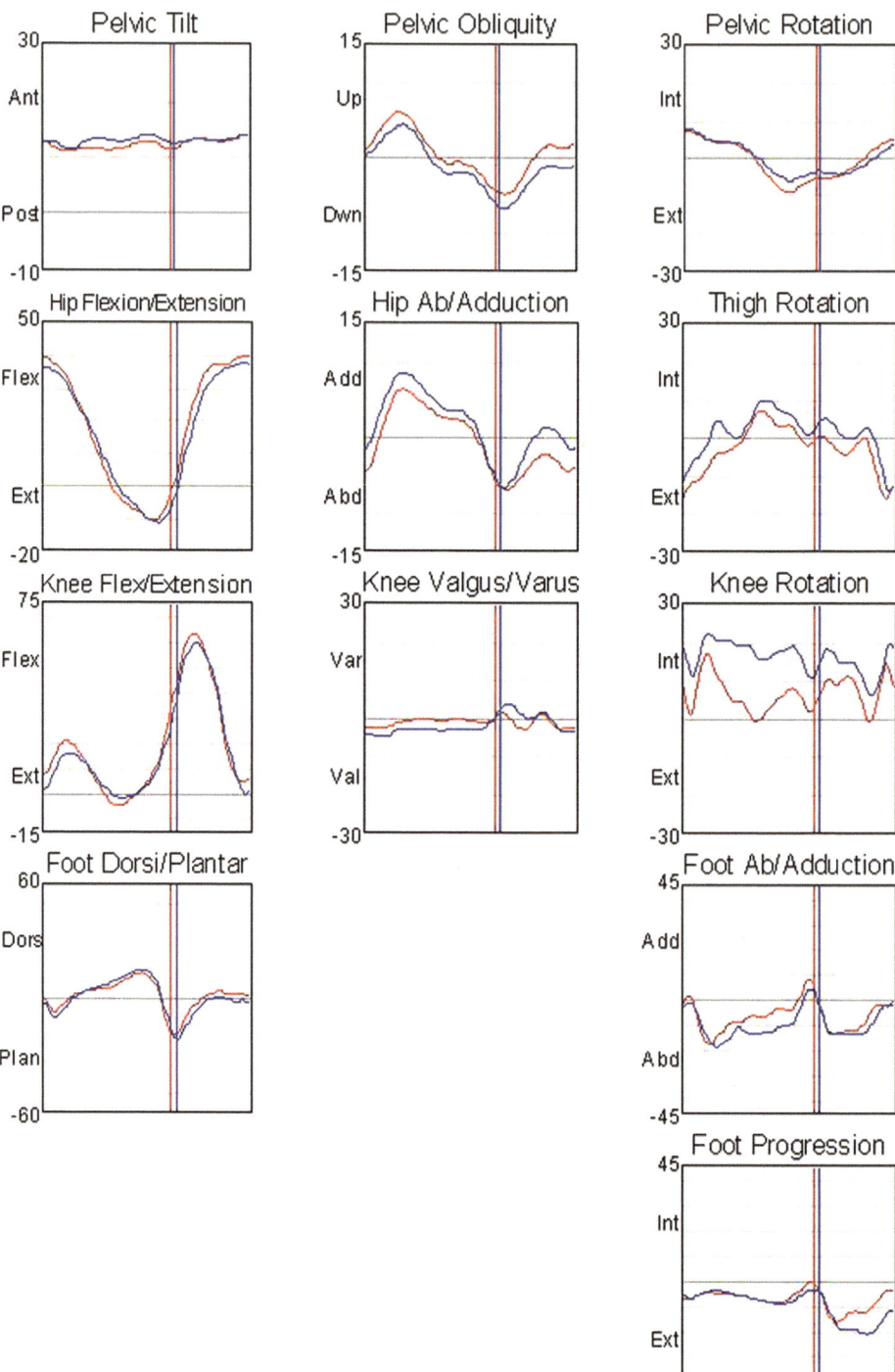

Energy Consumption

Energy consumption during walking indicates the efficiency of gait. Increased consumption suggests an inefficient gait and may contribute to the indications for treatment. Changes in energy consumption which follow treatment are clearly clinically relevant.

Energy consumption is judged indirectly by measuring oxygen consumption. This requires portable equipment to record the exhaled oxygen concentration. In addition, the carbon dioxide produced can be measured. In the absence of sophisticated equipment, the physiological cost index (PCI) of gait can be measured:

$$PCI = (\text{heart rate during walking} - \text{resting heart rate})/\text{speed}.$$

This has been shown to be a reliable indicator of gait energy efficiency.

Plantar Pressure and Foot Kinematics

Information about foot function while walking often helps in planning treatment. State-of-the-art pedobarographs describe the distribution of pressure over the plantar surface of the foot throughout the gait cycle. In recent years the increasing accuracy and resolution of equipment have allowed the development of kinematic foot models. These allow assessment of the motion between different moving segments of the foot during walking. Validation of these models in children is necessary before their clinical use is implemented [5]. Moreover, this information can be synchronized with the kinematic data to allow gait events to be married to changes in plantar pressure [6].

Clinical Application of Gait Analysis

The clinical use of gait analysis was first established in managing children with cerebral palsy [1, 3]. The complex patterns of walking in these children, the interaction between problems in different joints and muscles, and the unpredictability of results following orthopaedic surgery led to the development of motion analysis laboratories. With the support of gait analysis, the concept of single-stage, multi-level orthopaedic surgery replaced the multiple isolated procedures performed year by year and described as the "birthday syndrome" by Mercer Rang [7]. New procedures were developed or refined with the improved understanding of gait abnormalities [8–10]. Currently, most centers managing children with cerebral palsy use gait analysis as part of their preoperative planning of single-stage, multi-level surgery in diplegia as well as in the more complex forms of hemiplegia. Despite some continuing controversy on the repeatability of gait data interpretation, there is evidence that the proper use of gait analysis has led to better results [11].

Gait analysis has also been used extensively in myelodysplasia [12]. Detection of excessive valgus knee strain (valgus thrust) and discrimination between coronal and transverse plane deviations, particularly around the hip, are often the indications for analysis. For example, the combination of dynamic internal hip rotation and external tibial torsion seen in patients with lumbar myelomeningocoele may be mistaken for valgus knee. Transverse plane kinematic data reveal any dynamic rotation while walking, while coronal plane data reveal any valgus knee strain. The differentiation between these two problems is important in management.

Kinematic and kinetic analyses often guide the indications for various orthotics and their modifications to optimize the effects of the ground reaction force. Dynamic spasticity of the plantarflexors persisting throughout the gait cycle may need a rigid ankle foot orthosis (AFO), while equinus in swing may be treated with a flexible AFO which allows dorsiflexion. A ground reaction AFO may help when spasticity of the plantarflexors prevents full knee extension in stance.

Furthermore, after fitting orthoses, gait analysis may be used to tune them. For example, a tendency to knee hyperextension may be managed by pitching an AFO forward by raising the heel. Incomplete knee extension can be treated by pitching the AFO posteriorly and transferring the ground reaction force forward. The video vector technique (video with the ground reaction force superimposed) can be used for this purpose.

Gait analysis, particularly kinetics, may help to resolve treatment dilemmas for common anatomical variants. Genu valgum or varum, in-toeing due to persistent femoral anteversion, internal tibial torsion, or metatarsus adductus, as well as out-toeing due to external hip rotation or tibial torsion are common problems in paediatric orthopaedic clinics. When these normal variants persist beyond the expected remodeling age, a decision has to be made as to whether surgical correction is necessary. In mild cases gait analysis can offer reassurance by demonstrating the absence of any abnormal forces and moments in the proximal joints. With significant anatomical deviation, kinetic abnormalities will be present. This may provide a relative indication for treatment, as abnormal moments may pre-dispose to premature joint degeneration in adult life.

Conclusion

In recent years, several clinical studies on children with orthopaedic problems have used gait analysis as an outcome measure (e.g., congenital club foot, Perthes disease, and end-stage hip arthropathy requiring arthrodesis) [13–15]. These studies underline the importance of assessing gait before and after treatment, particularly when walking ability is the main indication for treatment. By assessing objectively the results of treatment better outcomes should follow. The possibilities for using gait analysis in children with orthopaedic conditions are enormous.

There are promising improvements in gait analysis technology on the horizon. Improved accuracy, speedier acquisition, and strict clinical protocols will improve repeatability. Better biomechanical models and custom-specific models will allow us to combine gait analysis with imaging techniques such as MRI. Forward simulation techniques will permit the creation of biomechanical models where surgery and its outcomes may be simulated before definitive treatment.

References

1. Gage JR. The treatment of gait problems in cerebral palsy series: clinics in developmental medicine, No. 164. London: Mac Keith Press, 2004.

2. Hof AL. Scaling gait data to body size. Gait Posture 1996; 4: 222–3.
3. Sutherland D. The development of mature gait. Gait Posture 1997; 6: 163–70.
4. Read HS, Hazlewood ME, Hillman SJ, et al. Edinburgh visual gait score for use in cerebral palsy. 2003; 23(3):296–301.
5. Stebbins J, Harrington M, Thompson N, et al. Repeatability of a model for measuring foot kinematics in children. Gait Posture 2006; 23(4):401–10.
6. Stebbins J, Harrington M, Giacomozzi C, et al. Assessment of subdivision of plantar pressure measurement in children. Gait Posture 2005; 22(4):372–6.
7. Wenger DR, Rang M. The art and practice of children's orthopaedics. New York: Raven Press; 1993.
8. Ounpuu S, Muik E, Davis RB 3rd, et al. Rectus femoris surgery in children with cerebral palsy. Part II: A comparison between the effect of transfer and release of the distal rectus femoris on knee motion. J Pediatr Orthop 1993; 13(3):331–5.
9. Seniorou M, Thompson N, Harrington M, Theologis T. Recovery of muscle strength following multi-level orthopaedic surgery in diplegic cerebral palsy. Gait Posture 2007; 26(4):475–81.
10. Lee CL, Bleck EE. Surgical correction of equinus deformity in cerebral palsy. Dev Med Child Neurol 1980; 22(3):287–92.
11. Graham HK, Harvey A. Assessment of mobility after multi-level surgery for cerebral palsy. J Bone Joint Surg Br 2007; 89(8):993–4.
12. Duffy CM, Hill AE, Cosgrove AP, et al. Three-dimensional gait analysis in spina bifida. J Pediatr Orthop 1996; 16(6):786–91.
13. Westhoff B, Petermann A, Hirsch MA, et al. Computerized gait analysis in Legg Calvé Perthes disease—analysis of the frontal plane. Gait Posture 2006; 24(2):196–202.
14. Karol LA, Halliday SE, Gourineni P. Gait and function after intra-articular arthrodesis of the hip in adolescents. J Bone Joint Surg Am 2000; 82(4):561–9.
15. Theologis TN, Harrington ME, Thompson N, Benson MK. Dynamic foot movement in children treated for congenital talipes equinovarus. J Bone Joint Surg Br 2003; 85(4):572–7.

Chapter 2

Neuromotor Development and Examination

Robert A. Minns

Introduction

The adult nervous system is essentially a *static system* (or one which is in decline) and the clinical neurological examination is therefore cross-sectional. The paediatric neurologist, however, has to examine all of the various pathways of the nervous system, mindful of the timing of the appearance (and disappearance) of various developmental signs.

Most signs that are abnormal to the adult neurologist may, at some stage of development, be normal in the fetus and infant. For example, all of the signs that accompany an acute hemiplegic stroke in the adult can be normal in a healthy newborn baby. All infants have features of a double hemiplegia including apraxia, grasp reflex, brisk phasic reflexes, ankle clonus, and extensor plantar responses with extrapyramidal-type progression movement or neonatal athetoid movements. In a child with a later dense hemiplegia, no clinical abnormalities may be evident during the neonatal period; the neurological asymmetries and deficits develop later, so that by 3–5 years of age there are overt signs of a dense hemiplegia.

Similarly, at 13 months, when the child takes his or her first independent steps, the gait is broad based, the arms are held out from the side, and foot placement is pronated. This is really a physiological ataxia.

A number of clinical features are seen in normal children which, in the adolescent or adult would be regarded as representing neurological abnormality, but which are purely a reflection of maturation of the nervous system. These *maturational* (previously called "soft") *signs* in 6–8-year-olds include "mirror movements" to the opposite limb (arm to arm or arm to leg) and associated movements (opening the mouth or shoulder and elbow movements) in 52% of normal children; mirror dyspraxia (building blocks in reverse

fashion) occur in 13%; finger agnosia in 29%; inaccurate graphesthesia in 46%; ambilaterality (changing hands for the same and different tasks) in 23%; poor cross commands in 26% dynamic gesturing difficulties in 26%; and right–left discrimination in 9% [1].

Therefore it is important to not only be able to elicit these signs but to know the "plus and minus two standard deviations" of when they appear and disappear as a means of recognizing the pathological.

Brain Development

Brain development underpins all neurodevelopment and determines the effect of brain insults, occurring from early intrauterine life to approximately 5 years of age. Developmental assessment therefore depends upon the orderly programmed rate and sequence of brain development.

Stages of brain development include

1. Formation of the neural crest and closure of the neural tube. The neural folds and neural groove become evident at 22 days post-conception. Fusion of the neural tube commences in the middle of the neural fold and proceeds to "zip up" simultaneously in both proximal and distal directions. The proximal closure (anterior neuropore) is complete at 26 days and the rostral (posterior neuropore) at 28–30 days. By 21 days post-conception, cells at the side of the neural plate and normal ectoderm form the neural crest. Abnormalities at this stage result in neural tube defects (myelomeningocele and anencephaly), Arnold–Chiari malformation, Danny–Walker malformation, and caudal regression syndrome.

2. Primitive vesicle formation. The proximal neural tube dilates at about 28 days into three primitive vesicles: the prosencephalon, the mesencephalon, and the rhombencephalon. With lengthening, the cervical and

R.A. Minns (✉)
Department of Child Life and Health, University of Edinburgh, Edinburgh, UK; Royal Hospital for Sick Children, Edinburgh, UK

pontine flexures occur. Abnormalities include holopros-encephaly, absence of corpus callosum, and septo-optic dysplasia.

3. Division of the telencephalon. The prosencephalon divides into the telencephalon and diencephalon. The telencephalon gives rise to the cortex. The telencephalon and the diencephalon give rise to the thalamus and the basal ganglia and the diencephalon also gives rise to the hypothalamus. The mesencephalon forms the mid-brain and the rhombencephalon the cerebellum, pons, and medulla. Each primitive division further divides into neuromeres under specific genetic control.

4. Cell division. Primitive stem cells arise in the germi-nal matrix adjacent to the ependyma of the telencephalic vesicle where they divide into two. One of these primi-tive neuroblasts will migrate and the other will continue to produce several generations of clone cells.

5. Cell migration along Bergmann fibers. Programmed neuroblasts migrate along invisible glial processes (Bergmann glial fibers) to form the future cortex. The cell migrates according to the "inside out rule" where the more recently migrating cell is more exter-nal. Cell division in the subependymal region remains active upto 28 weeks. Most neurones have migrated by 20 weeks and subsequently glioblasts (glial pre-cursors) migrate. With increasing cell numbers the previously smooth cerebral cortex before 22 weeks now infolds with gyral formation. Abnormalities at this stage include cortical dysplasias, neurofibromato-sis, tuberous sclerosis, effects of cocaine addiction, Zellweger syndrome, fetal alcohol syndrome, and lissencephaly.

6. Axonal and dendritic development. There are six dif-ferent neurone types in the cortex and they require to be correctly orientated, i.e., axons pointing downward. Connections are probably induced by chemical attrac-tants. Dendritic growth is maximal from 28 to 35 weeks with the formation of dendritic spines. Glial multiplica-tion (from 28 to 40 weeks) is responsible for the second DNA spurt.

7. Apoptosis. Redundant processes with no synaptic con-tact will dissolve; between 28 and 34 weeks the subependymal zone (germinal plate) undergoes rapid dissolution.

8. Synaptic pruning.

9. Angiogenesis.

10. Myelination. Myelin is produced by the oligodendroglial cells in the central nervous system and by Schwann cells in the peripheral nervous system. Each oligodendroglial cell can myelinate up to 15 axons. This allows rapid conduction down the axon and insulation from the ionic changes in the extracellular environment. As the brain weighs 350 g at birth and 1350 g at 4 years, much of this increase is due to myelination and the formation of dendrites, Nissl granules, and association pathways. It occurs rapidly in the first 6 months after birth, at a slower phase over the next 4 years, and then very slowly up to 16 years. Abnormalities at this stage include delayed myelination and dysmyelination.

11. Association fiber development. There are definite myel-ogenetic cycles [2]. The leg area of the cortex myelinates before the arm region, yet upper limb function is in advance of walking. Myelination of short association pathways such as the fronto-hypothalamic tract occurs during the first 12 years of life. These inhibit the nor-mal inhibitory pathway from the habenular nucleus to the pituitary, allowing puberty to develop. Association pathways are important for mental functions.

12. Dominance. The left side of the brain, particularly over the superior aspect of the temporal lobe, is anatomi-cally different from the right, with many more cells and with preprogramming for the learning of language. If a module is damaged on one side of the brain it can be taken over by the opposite lobe. Normally one side is inhibited, producing reciprocal cerebral inhibition or dominance so that there is no interference between one side of the brain and the other. These stages of devel-opment include the primary areas such as the motor strip, somatosensory and visual areas, and Heschl's gyrus.

13. Maturation of tertiary areas. Secondary association areas for vision, Wernicke's area, and motor association areas have connections across the corpus callosum and long intracortical connections. Maturation of the angular gyrus and frontal pole are the last to mature.

14. Psychogenesis. By this is meant the effect of the envi-ronment on brain development before and after birth. Prior to birth cerebral nutritive factors are paramount and following birth the external environment influ-ences development. The basic items of development (sitting, standing, walking, and crawling) are geneti-cally determined and therefore not learned or influenced by environment. However, the developmental skills are certainly influenced by environment, learning through walking, and in turn how to run, hop, skip, jump, and so on. Examples of this include infants in certain cultures who are swaddled until well into the second year of life. Since walking occurs within a few days of removal of the swaddling, nurture has been rather overstated with respect to these basic items of develop-ment. Adverse environmental influences, when reversed, can result in "catch up." For example, the previously institutionalized child shows quite retarded development emotionally and in speech and language but less retar-dation in the areas of posture and movement. When the child is removed to an optimal environment these

previously delayed items show "catch up." Measured intelligence may rise and brain size increase to the point of even splitting the cranial sutures. In severe psycho-social deprivation brain growth ceases, producing the clinical appearances of deprivation dwarfism. The child is floppy, pot-bellied, and manifests with poor visual and auditory responses along with poor responses to painful stimuli. Adrenocorticotropic hormones (ACTH) and growth hormone are low, giving the appearance of panhypopituitarism. Experimental animals stimulated through one eye only show increased myelination in the ipsilateral optic nerves. The practice of nursing a young infant prone results in earlier acquisition of crawling but no other developmental milestones. On the negative side, however, such babies often present with persistent toe walking. Babies nursed supine exclusively adopt a more "cowboy" pattern of ambulation.

15. Senescence.

Principles of Development Testing

Maturation is tested in young children by combining functional assessments of developmental items into groups such as gross motor skills (also called posture and mobility or locomotor); manipulation and vision; hearing, speech, and language; and social and emotional behavior.

Although all are functional items (e.g., reaching out for objects) they all involve many neurological pathways. Milestones reflect the acquisition of skills consequent upon neurodevelopmental maturation.

To commence an understanding of the neurodevelopmental examination one can build on the adult neurological examination which assesses muscle power, tone, coordination and truncal balance, phasic reflexes, sensation, cranial nerves, and higher cortical function. Posture and movement (as above) will therefore be assessing muscle power and tone.

Subcortical integrators of posture and movement are called "primitive reflexes," and in conditions where there is a delay or abnormality in posture and movement development these primitive reflexes persist.

Manipulation similarly involves pathways of muscle power, coordination, and praxic ability. Cranial nerves II–VI are concerned with vision, IX–XII with bulbar or feeding function, and VIII with acoustic and labyrinthine activity.

Social development requires conditioned learning rather than innate or cognitive learning; emotional development along with language represents aspects of higher cortical function. Speech is purely a motor act (articulation, phonation, and rhythm).

Major Influences on Development

Brain Damage

Acquired brain damage in the adult will result in hard neurological deficits such as hemiplegia, cortical blindness, and epilepsy. A similar insult to the developing brain not only results in these deficits but produces subsequent slowing of brain development either globally or focally. In general, global brain insults result in global delay and localized insults in specific delays. Acute system diseases have little effect upon the development of the nervous system but acute neurological disorders (affecting the organ of development) may produce substantial neurodevelopmental consequences. Chronic disease will retard optimal somatic growth but chronic neurological disease will impair neurological development as in chronic under-nutrition or hypothyroidism.

Gender

Males are delayed compared to females of a similar chronological age, presumably due to the retarding effect of the Y chromosome. Noxious influences at any particular time in development will therefore have more profound effects on the male, having the more immature nervous system.

Genetic Factors

Brain development is under genetic control and any ability would be expected to follow a normal distribution curve. Brain development continues until 17 or 18 years; however, the quicker the rate of early development, the earlier will be the completion of brain growth and development. Normal children who walk at 9 months will be no more proficient than those who walk at 14 months, and similarly with pubertal onset. In general fast achievers with a rapid rate of brain development ceiling earlier but do not continue with brain development for a longer period. Many developmental disorders such as dyslexia are proven to be genetic disorders and are not simply a slowing up of the normal rate of development (less than the third centile) because the deficit persists for life. It is important to differentiate a normal child with a slow rate of brain development from a developmental genetic disease or pathological brain insult slowing down brain development.

In general adverse genetic influences acting early in intrauterine life result in severe deficits such as anencephaly or spina bifida while those acting later affect migration and produce disorders such as tuberous sclerosis. Genetic deviants will be referred to later.

Neurodevelopment Examination (Concentrating on Posture and Movement/Mobility)

Figure 2.1 shows the normal development of posture and movement. It is essential to think of development in a longitudinal sense and not cross-sectionally, considering it from the most primitive through to the most normal. We have concentrated here on posture and movement/mobility because of the importance of this in orthopaedics although other aspects of development, manipulation, vision, hearing, speech, and language should also be considered in a longitudinal sense. The figure shows, at 12 weeks gestation, the first flexor phase of development, approximating to that of a spinal level. At 28 weeks a fetus is extended and this is equivalent to a lower

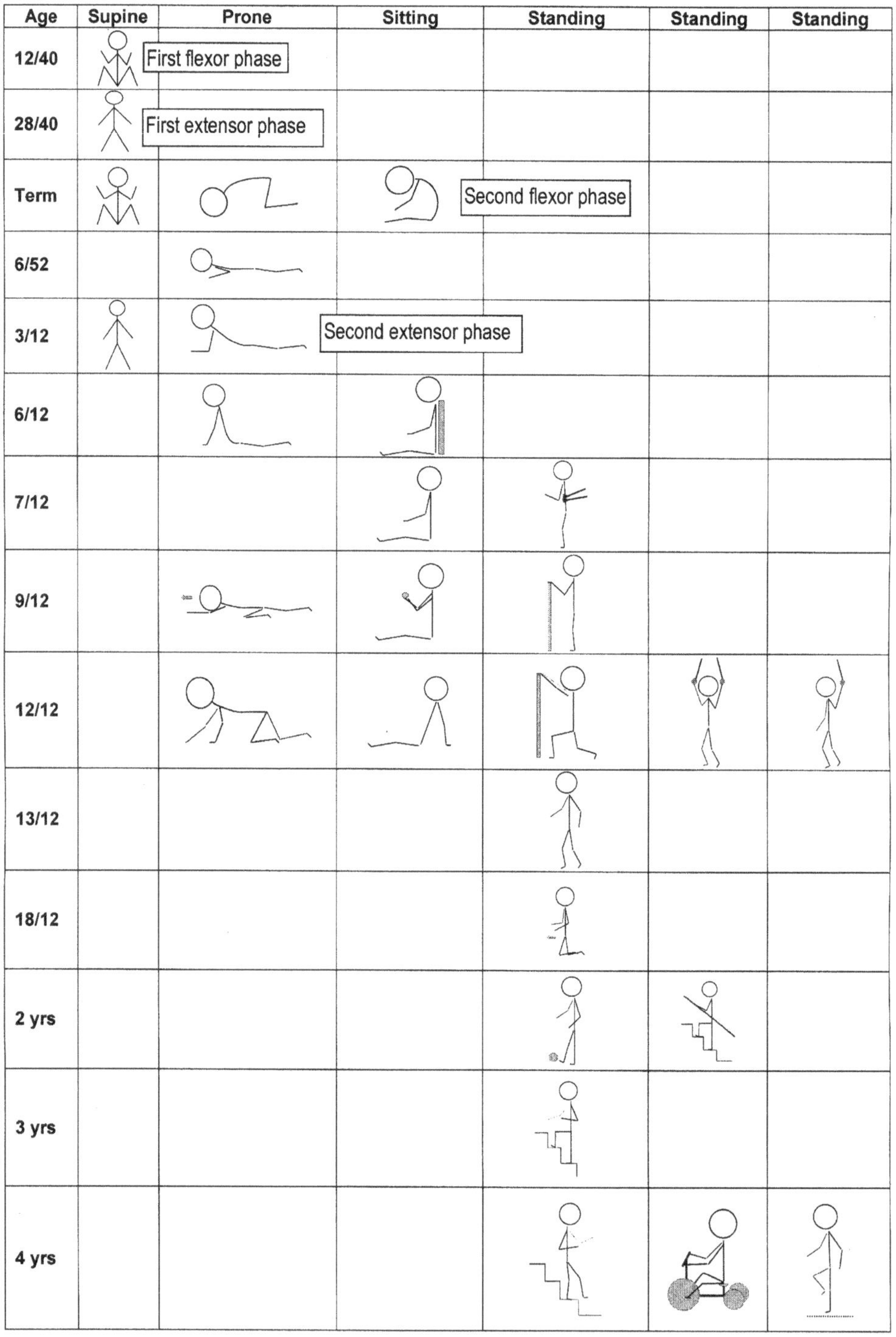

Age	Supine	Prone	Sitting	Standing	Standing	Standing
12/40		First flexor phase				
28/40		First extensor phase				
Term				Second flexor phase		
6/52						
3/12			Second extensor phase			
6/12						
7/12						
9/12						
12/12						
13/12						
18/12						
2 yrs						
3 yrs						
4 yrs						

Fig. 2.1 Schematic depiction of neuromotor development

brain stem level of functioning. The flexed term baby is functioning at a midbrain level. Thus the normal newborn has an impassive face with reptilian stare, quasi-athetoid hand movements, and oro-facial dyskinesia, which in the mature brain could indicate parkinsonism. By 3 months the baby is again in the second extensor phase where now, with cortical maturation, there is inhibition of lower centers. This changing pattern of first and second flexor and extensor phases does not represent a "change of mind" but rather increasing levels of hierarchical maturation.

In practical terms the infant's posture and movement are best assessed by looking at the child in four standard positions—supine, prone, sitting, and standing—first describing the posture that the child adopts and then the movements that he undertakes. After initial observations when supine, the child is pulled to sit (a traction response) and the degree of head lag or control is observed. The child is then observed in a sitting position. Again the child is pulled to stand and the posture and movements observed. Finally the child is placed prone by rotating the child through 180° (Fig. 2.2).

As the posture reflects tone and the movements reflect power this is truly a neurological assessment of a longitudinal (maturing) nervous system. Until 12 months of age the neurodevelopmental examination should consists of all these positions, but after 12 months all subsequent development of posture and movement occurs in the standing or vertical position.

When beginning to walk unaided, the infant frequently falls but immediately gets up and carries on and does this repeatedly. This is probably genetically "forced": there is a compulsion to use new developmental milestones when they come "on stream" to ensure that they are used. This is seen also in "forced grasping" at 3–4 months, forced visual pursuit, and forced utterances in early verbal communication.

These processes for learning skills must be differentiated from the appearance of basic items of development. For example, many of the later items of posture and movements/mobility *are* "true skills" and show a considerable variability in their age of acquisition in different developmental tests. Clearly the skills require the appropriate environment in order to advance.

Skills therefore depend upon the opportunity to practice and a lack of such skills in developmental histories should be carefully interpreted in the light of opportunity.

The learning of skills follows a very constant path, whether this is riding a bicycle, playing a piece of music on the piano, or learning to drive a car:

1. The movements are undertaken first in isolation.
2. They are made to involve both hands in sequence.
3. Speed is added to the skill.
4. When motor learning is complete and placed in the subconscious, dominant hemisphere expression takes over, producing fluidity of the skill with modulation from the non-dominant hemisphere.

Motor skills pathways involve the cerebellar hemispheres, red nucleus, dorsal nucleus, ophthalamus, motor strip, and premotor strip. The inability to sequence individual motor acts into a skill is *dyspraxia* and this is an abnormality which is an executive disorder of movement in the absence of hard neurological signs, producing clumsiness and an inability to learn certain skills. Praxis is necessary for skills involving movements of all types, not just gross motor skills. Similarly, dyspraxia may be seen as an axial dyspraxia, oculomotor dyspraxia, articulatory dyspraxia, ideomotor or ideational dyspraxia, or writing dyspraxia (dysgraphia). While many children of primary school age are reported to be clumsy, few adults admit to this because of subsequent maturation and also because, if there is a specific dyspraxic learning difficulty, the adult finds ways around this particular difficulty to achieve the task.

The progression in development in general occurs in a cephalocaudal direction and from mass function to discrete function, so that in the upper limb development proceeds from the shoulder first and then to the hand. Any diminution in function from a brain insult will result in a loss in the opposite direction, thus the hand is first involved. This

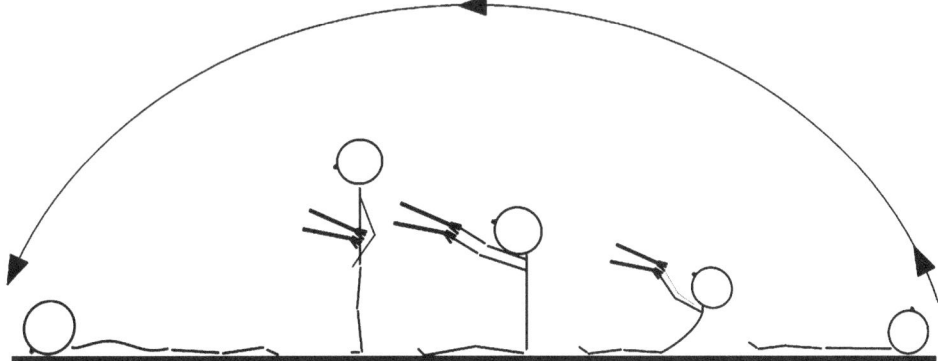

Fig. 2.2 Practical assessment of infant's posture and movements, through 180° change of position (including traction response)

can be seen, for example, with distal, severe praxic, and paralytic loss with the retention of proximal "fly-swatting" movements.

Until a new task becomes automatic it does require close attention by the child with sometimes an apparent lull in development of other areas. For example, at the commencement of independent walking upper limb function may appear to decline and thus one sees "fits and starts" in development.

Deviant Locomotor Development

Most children progress through posture and movement milestones in a common sequence: sitting, crawling, standing, and walking. However, 9% of the population are genetic deviants who have changed the order of this sequence. They frequently have an essential hypotonia, and this genetic trait is inherited in a dominant fashion. There are three distinct categories:

1. *Shufflers*, who represent 7% of the population. Their early motor milestones are delayed and they are hypotonic,

shuffling on their bottoms rather than crawling in a standard way. They sit alone at 10 months, "shuffle" (i.e., are mobile) at 12 months, and walk alone at 19 months.
2. *Rollers* constitute 1% of children and they are mobile mostly by rolling but do crawl very briefly before walking. They are also hypotonic and roll at $8\frac{1}{2}$ months, sit at 9 months, and walk unaided at 16 months.
3. *Creepers* form approximately 1% of the population and sit at 10 months, creep in a commando crawling fashion at $12\frac{1}{2}$ months, and walk at about 20 months.

It is thought that there are two groups of children here, those who crawl and those who do not. Those who crawl and have normal muscle tone are the standard crawlers of the population. Those who crawl with hypotonia are the rollers and creepers. Children who do not crawl and are hypotonic are the shufflers and those who do not crawl and have normal muscle tone are the "fast" deviants in the population.

Clearly, "shuffle trait," which is inherited, can accompany acquired brain damage, probably altering the acquisition of some milestones. Its effect on pre-existing spasticity is not really known. Shuffle trait is frequently seen in children with Down's and other syndromes. The importance of this to the

Table 2.1 Primitive reflexes

Reflex	Elicitation
Cranial nerve reflexes, e.g.	
Rooting	Stimulus to the cheek results in the head and mouth turning to the stimulus
Sucking	Insertion of a teat in the mouth
Startle	1. Sudden noise or tapping elicits a similar response to Moro (see below), except the elbows and hands remain flexed
Extensor reflexes, e.g.	
Asymmetrical tonic neck reflex	Present from 1 to 3 months; on turning the child's head to one side, the child adopts a "fencing posture" with extension of both limbs on the side turned to
Moro	From 29 weeks onwards; the infant is held supine facing the examiner and the head is allowed to drop back (controlled) with resultant:
	(i) brief adduction of arms
	(ii) extension of arms with hands open
	(iii) adduction of arms
Progression reflexes, e.g.	
Walking	With the infant in a vertical position and the feet touching the surface, tilting the child results in high stepping
Placing	Stimulation of the dorsum of the foot on the edge of the table causes flexion of the leg and then extension and placement on the surface
Cutaneous reflexes, e.g.	
Palmar grasp	Introducing a finger into the palm from the ulnar side causes finger flexion
Plantar grasp	Stroking the plantar surface of the digits results in their flexion. This response is elicited in both hands and feet from 16 weeks' gestation to 3 months postnatally.

physician is the recognition of a normal genetic deviant, thus avoiding invasive investigations (muscle enzyme, muscle biopsy, and neurophysiology) and allowing parents to be reassured of eventual normality.

Primitive Reflexes

The mature child and adolescent can change posture and movements independently (e.g., can sit and write, lie prone and write, stand and write). The young infant, however, is unable to do so and there are subcortical integrators of posture and movement which ensure that if the child is placed in a certain position he will adopt a certain movement or posture. For example, the supine infant whose head is turned to one side will adopt a fencing posture. This is a *primitive reflex*. Some 70 or more of these have been described but should be considered as only one small facet of the neurodevelopmental examination of the infant. They can be grouped as cranial nerve primitive reflexes, extensor primitive reflexes, progression primitive reflexes, and cutaneous primitive reflexes. The important and easily recognizable progression reflexes are shown in Table 2.1.

These primitive reflexes are present early in development and disappear with maturation at a variable time. When brain insult causes cerebral palsy, by definition an abnormality of posture and movement due to an unchanging or static brain damage occurring during the period of brain growth or due to a congenital malformation of the brain, the integrators of posture and movement (primitive reflexes) persist, sometimes for life. Certain types of cerebral palsy are more frequently seen with persistent primitive reflexes. Their presence, however (e.g., primitive swimming reflex), does not signify potential future Olympic athletes.

Phasic Reflexes

Phasic reflexes must be differentiated from primitive reflexes. They are routinely assessed in the neurological examination and their absence signifies an interruption of the spinal reflex with denervation of either the afferent or the efferent pathway. Myopathic disorders with stretch receptors involved, or with severe myopathic weakness, will also result in reduced or absent phasic reflexes.

They are considerably uninhibited in infants compared to older children and are frequently elicited by means of a finger tap rather than conventional tendon hammer at that age. These reflexes are important in delineating neurosegmental levels in spinal cord lesions such as transverse myelitis or in

myelomeningocele. Their innervation is essential to know: ankle jerks S1–2 and knee jerks L3–4.

Signs of a pathological brisk phasic reflex include

- exaggerated response
- small amplitude stimulus
- wide afferent field
- crossed adduction
- clonus

A few beats of clonus are normal in early infancy. An extensor plantar response (Babinski sign) does not indicate pyramidal dysfunction and will normally be extensor until 12 months of age. Rarely, a flexor plantar response will be a false-negative finding with other signs of pyramidal dysfunction in the older child. Tendon reflexes in the upper limbs are normally less brisk than those in the lower limbs when elicited in a sitting position.

Examination of an infant or young child will often be less threatening and ensure more compliance if the child is examined sitting on the mother's lap and without the exposure of a tendon hammer.

Muscle Power

Movement reflects power and may be observed generally, although individual muscle groups often require an assessment of power in a more quantified way. The Medical Research Council (MRC) [3] developed the following scale:

0 = complete paralysis
1 = a flicker of contraction
2 = muscle can make normal movement with gravity eliminated
3 = normal movement against gravity but not additional resistance
4 = full normal power but overcome by resistance
5 = normal power

In the newborn it is important to distinguish hypotonia from weakness by observing volitional movement when the child is stimulated remote from the limbs (i.e., nose and anterior chest) and noting the resultant limb movements or crying or sucking.

There is an inherent relationship between muscle power and function in that a patient needs quadriceps power greater than MRC 3 for stance and good psoas activity for hip flexion during walking.

Proximal power in the upper limbs is assessed quickly and functionally by asking the child to raise the arms above the head, to touch the back of the neck, to stretch out the hands at the side, and to touch the base of the spine, the opposite knee, or hip. Distal power in the upper limb is readily assessed by grasp, finger abduction and adduction, and attempting to break opposition of thumb and index finger.

Muscle Tone Assessment

Muscle tone is a reflection of posture as mentioned above. It is assessed in quite discrete ways: by measuring resistance to passive movements, estimation of the joint angles, the feel of the muscles themselves, and by the posture.

1. Resistance to passive movements is generally assessed at the elbows, hips, knees, ankles, and wrists.
2. Joint angles are assessed clinically (rather than by using objective means such as goniometers) based upon a knowledge of the normal range of joint motion at different chronological ages:

   a. The elbow is assessed from a zero starting position with the arm straight; since this is a hinge joint natural movement is in flexion. Motion beyond the zero starting position is an unnatural one and is referred to as hyperextension. This may be evident in hypotonic children and is usually assessed in degrees beyond the zero starting point.
   b. Forearm pronation and supination are assessed from a vertical, zero starting, or "thumbs up" position with the forearms at the side of the body and the elbows flexed to 90°. Pronation ranges from 0 to 90° and supination from 0 to 90°. Excessive supination may enable the child to place the dorsum of his hands together when holding the arms extended and supinated (Fig. 2.3).

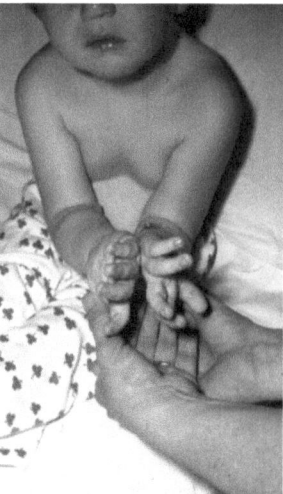

Fig. 2.3 Demonstrating hypersupination with elbows almost extended, indicative of exaggerated joint angles and hypotonia

i. Radial/ulnar deviations are not usually used for joint angle assessment of muscle tone, but the fingers of the hands are occasionally used.
ii. The *thumb* has a number of complex movements including abduction, adduction, flexion, extension, and opposition (circumduction). Extension of the thumb is undertaken parallel to the plane of the palm and is normally 90°. When it is excessive the thumb approximates to the radial forearm.
iii. The wrist may also be used as an indicator, particularly of hypotonia, with the forearm held upright and the hand allowed to fall forward. The hand normally makes an angle of 30° with the horizontal plane through the wrist. This is considerably less in hypotonic states (Holmes' sign) [4].

c. The shoulder has an almost complete range of global motion and indicators of hypotonia here are the "scarf sign," with the arms wrapped around the chest and the position of the olecranon assessed in relation to the nipple line (Fig. 2.4). In hypotonic states the elbows may approximate posteriorly. On lifting a hypotonic child under the axillae the examiner's hands may "slip through" the shoulder joint.
d. The spine may be assessed for exaggerated joint angles by looking at the degree of forward flexion and converting that angle to a measured distance such as inches from the floor to the fingertips, or in lateral movements of the spine, the distance the fingertips descend along the thigh.
e. The "straight leg raising" test, although not a record of spine motion, is carried out with the child lying supine on a firm, level examining table. The upward movement of the straight leg is a passive motion and measured in degrees from the zero starting position. The two sides may be compared (for more details, see Chapter 19).
f. The hip, which is a ball and socket joint, has a lesser range of motion than the shoulder. From a zero position and with the opposite leg held in maximum flexion (by the examiner or patient), thus flattening the lumbar spine, any hip flexion deformity of the other hip is demonstrated (Thomas' test). The examiner should place one hand on the iliac crest to note the point at which the pelvis begins to rotate. The normal range of active hip flexion is 110–120° [5]. Passive flexion may be as much as 140°+. Hip rotation in flexion and in extension is measured in angles. This gives an estimate of femoral anteversion, a cause for intoeing (along with diplegia and tibial torsion). Abduction and adduction of the normal hip are 45° and 40°, respectively, with knees extended and 45–60° with the knees flexed.

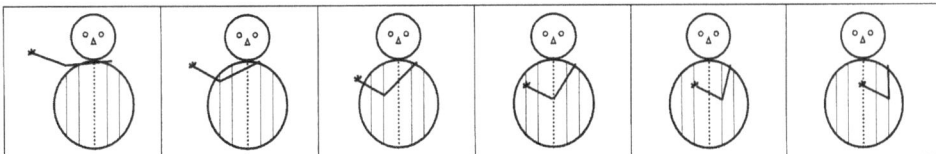

Fig. 2.4 The scarf sign is assessed by bringing one arm across the infant's chest until resistance is met. It tests passive tone in the flexors of the shoulder girdle. With increasing maturity (from 28 to 37 weeks post-conception or hypotonia) the elbow reaches from (i) the neck, (ii) opposite axillary line, (iii) opposite nipple line, (iv) xiphoid process, (v) ipsilateral nipple line, and (vi) ipsilateral axillary line

g. The knee is a modified hinge joint and the primary motion is flexion. It is examined looking for hyperextension and excessive flexion (i.e., greater than 135°). The "popliteal angle" is a useful joint angle particularly in newborns.

h. The ankle is another modified hinge joint, flexion, and extension occurring at the tibiotalar joint. It also has a slight degree of lateral motion when the ankle is plantarflexed. The zero point here is with the leg at right angles to the thigh and the foot at right angles to the shin. There is normally some 50° of combined tibiotalar and subtalar plantar flexion and 20° of dorsiflexion. Average ranges of joint motion may be found in various texts such as that published by the American Academy of Orthopaedic Surgeons 1965 [5].

3. The feel of the muscle is a rather subjective assessment of muscle tone but is applicable in states of gross hyper- and hypotonicity.
4. Posture. The "pithed frog posture" or round shouldered (slouching) posture may indicate poor tone. When the patient is examined on a firm examining couch there will be multiple points of contact between the body and the bed (i.e., no normal curvatures are evident). Disordered posture may indicate hypo- or hypertonia. Abnormal postures include

- Squint baby syndrome
- "Windsweeping" deformity
- "W sitting"
- Transient dystonia of prematurity
- "Sitting in air" (an elemental sensorimotor pattern, not a primitive reflex)

Hypotonia

Hypotonia may be of central or peripheral origin. If of central origin there will be preservation or exaggeration of phasic reflexes which are absent or diminished with peripheral causes. Increased joint angles may be due to hypotonia but may also be due to congenital ligamentous laxity. In this situation the joint angles *do not* reflect a reduced muscle tone

as these individuals frequently do not have muscle hypotonia or weakness and may be contortionists or gymnasts. Various types of Ehlers–Danlos syndrome and congenital laxity of ligaments may give rise to a broad-based waddling gait, difficulty in rising from sitting, and an ability to assume abnormal postures such as placing the palms on the floor or make head-to-knee contact with knees extended. A further example of the ligamentous contribution to joint angles as a false-positive assessment of muscle tone can be demonstrated after a tendon lengthening for equinus deformity. No change in the muscle tone has been induced but the joint angle is increased. Likewise, exercise-induced muscle lengthening (the addition of sarcomeres) will result in some increase in joint angles.

In many conditions hypotonia and weakness may co-exist and in central core disease (a metabolic myopathy) hypotonia may be more obvious than weakness. With cerebellar hemisphere lesions abnormalities of coordination occur ipsilateral to the hemisphere involved with ipsilateral accompanying hypotonia. In the young infant with immature cerebellar and spinocerebellar pathways hypotonia may be the only sign of a cerebellar lesion. Ataxia must therefore enter the differential diagnosis of the "floppy baby."

The floppy infant will also present with delayed motor milestones and many severely learning disabled children are hypotonic.

Clinical Grades of Hypotonia

Hypotonia may be graded as follows:

0 = normal muscle tone
1 = decreased resistance to passive movement only
2 = decreased resistance to passive movement and joint hyperextensibility (i.e., increased joint angles)
3 = decreased resistance to passive movement and joint hyperextensibility causing postural effects in the lower limbs (e.g., valgus feet)
4 = decreased resistance to passive movement and joint hyperextensibility causing truncal postural effects (e.g., hyperlordosis)
5 = decreased resistance to passive movement and joint hyperextensibility causing postural effects in the shoulders and upper limbs (e.g., round shoulders)

Hypertonia

Spasticity is defined as stretch-dependent hypertonus which is abolished by posterior root section. There are two types, phasic and tonic. *Phasic spasticity* depends upon response to rapid stretch and is the earliest increase in muscle tone seen after cerebral lesions. This is often replaced with *tonic spasticity* which depends upon type 1 muscle fibers and does not vary with the velocity of stretch applied. The amount of lengthening of the muscle is reduced and the tonic muscle spindles fire for as long as the stretch is maintained. There is reciprocal inhibition of the antagonists and contractures occur in flexor, but not in the antigravity muscles. Tonic muscles are particularly geared to postural control. Occasionally there may be very little distal spasticity in combination with proximal tonic spasticity giving the appearance of a primary muscle disorder, the so-called proximal diplegia. In another group of children there is tonic paresis yet phasic spasticity with brisk reflexes, ankle clonus but a marked increase in muscle lengthening and joint ranges. This is often labeled ataxic diplegia or ataxic quadriplegia.

The original Ashworth Scale [6] is frequently used to assess increased muscle tone in adults:

1. No increase in muscle tone.
2. Slight increase in tone giving a "catch" when the affected part is moved in flexion or extension.
3. More marked increase in tone but the affected part is easily flexed.
4. Considerable increase in tone; passive movement difficult.
5. Affected part is rigid in flexion or extension.

Rigidity is an involuntary, sustained contraction of muscle but not muscle spindle dependent. It is driven by labyrinthine and proprioceptive systems and shows a constant resistance at varying angles. It is characterized by co-contraction of agonists and antagonists which may impose recognizably typical postures. There are two main types, *extensor dystonic rigidity* which produces clinical features depending upon whether there is labyrinthine or proprioceptive input which predominates. The muscle tone with rigidity is influenced by

1. contact with the surface
2. relationship of head to body
3. position in space
4. pressure through the long axis

The typical "prone/supine discrepancy" is an example of the dystonia seen in infancy from changing the head position. It is also influenced by anxiety, certain noises, lights, and esophageal reflux (Sandifer syndrome). These children have profuse primitive reflexes.

The second type is *flexor dystonia*. This is organized at the red nuclei/capsule. There are no progression or extensor reflexes in this pattern of deformity which is characterized by flexion at the arms, flexor recoil, and flexion of the legs but a normal lengthening reaction and a full range of movement. These types of deformity are therefore not fixed but dynamic deformities. These types of rigidity are clearly extrapyramidal and characteristically variable. They tend to affect all muscle groups—limb, axial, bulbar, and facial.

Mechanisms of Deformity in Children with Motor Disorders

The neurological examination attempts to understand the underlying mechanisms for the production of the dynamic, fixed, or structural deformity before the appropriate orthopaedic operation, drug, rhizotomy, or cerebellar stimulation. A further important fundamental is that positional deformities, whether intrauterine or postnatally acquired, may totally override the neurological picture which can make assessment of the etiology of the deformity difficult. Deformities may arise in several ways:

• Tonic spasticity
• Rigidity
• Paresis and muscle imbalance
• Growth
• Positional deformity
• Compensatory deformity
• Iatrogenic deformity
• Soft tissue contractural deformity
• Biomechanical muscle change

Positional deformities occur as a result of immobility plus the effect of growth and gravity. They may be seen in the neurologically normal child, in the neonatal physiological immobility of prematurity with resultant ballerina or cowboy postures, as mentioned previously, and in the "squint baby syndrome." They are seen in the neurologically abnormal child in its worst form with "wind sweeping," but also in "baby buggy spine" with knee flexion contractures from sitting in a wheelchair, and equinus feet from restrictive bed clothes covering the acutely ill child.

Contractures (to be distinguished from contractions) occur in many neurological conditions of childhood such as

1. Myopathies, especially:

   • Duchenne muscular dystrophy
   • Emery–Dreifuss sex-linked muscular dystrophy
   • Congenital fiber-type disproportion

2. Denervating conditions:

- Intermediate forms of chronic spinal muscular dystrophy
- Traumatic denervation
- Poliomyelitis
- Post-infective polyneuritis
- Prenatal denervation producing arthrogryposis

3. Spastic disorders:

- Cerebral palsy (hemiplegic, diplegic, and quadriplegic)
- Hereditary spastic diplegia

4. Extrapyramidal disorders:

- Athetoid/dystonic cerebral palsy
- Torsion dystonia
- Post-encephalitic athetosis
- Post-anoxic damage to the basal ganglia
- Genetically determined neurometabolic syndromes

Contractures may be dynamic (appearing during movement), fixed (independent of movement or immobility), and structural when secondary bone and joint changes have resulted from the persistent contracture.

Muscle Fasciculation

Muscle fasciculation, signifying lower motor denervation, is best seen in the tongue but also in the interossei along with fine, irregular tremor of the fingers in infants and young children with spinal muscular atrophy. Fasciculation may be elicited by tapping the muscle belly with the finger. It is seen particularly in the thenar and hypothenar muscles of the hand and in the shoulder muscles.

Muscle Wasting, Trophic, and Growth Changes

Muscle wasting or atrophy in childhood neurological conditions may result from central causes such as parietal (sensory) wasting in the affected limb and may also be due to trophic changes resulting from the autonomic dysfunction accompanying peripheral neuropathies. Other trophic effects will include changes to skin, hair, nails, and bone, characteristic of myelomeningocele, poliomyelitis, and arthrogryposis. Somatic growth changes frequently result from other generalized and functional limitations affecting feeding, weight bearing, and walking.

Muscle Wasting and Trophic Changes from Cerebral Lesions

Trophic limb changes may occur from a unilateral parietal lobe lesion. Aram et al. [7] found that there were corresponding contralateral shorter lengths of the hands and feet in children up to the age of 6 years who had no hemiplegia whereas there were no differences in normal children. If a unilateral brain lesion without hemiplegia can produce significant unilateral atrophy then this must at least contribute to the unilateral wasting in hemiplegia.

The pyramidal tract has a close relationship to the parapyramidal (autonomic) tracts which control vasomotor responses since movement inevitably requires an increase in blood flow to the muscle. Pyramidal lesions such as at the internal capsule or cortex can involve the parapyramidal tracts. This is evidenced by the fact that the wasted limb is often affected by abnormalities in vasomotor (vascular) control, with cold, blue limbs, prolonged capillary return, poor healing, and thickened nails.

Growth Failure in Cerebral Palsy and Other Neurological Conditions

In cerebral palsy the incidence of short stature and growth failure is high and the limbs are short and thin. This may be generalized in quadriplegic cerebral palsy with short stature (poor linear or skeletal growth) and wasting, or it may occur in a more localized fashion with a short limb (muscle and bone) that is thin (dwarfed or wasted) in hemiplegic or diplegic cerebral palsy.

In hemiplegia the disturbance is more likely to affect the leg than the arm and results in dwarfing of the lower limb or unequal leg lengths; a 2 cm difference between the lower limbs was found by Lin and Brown [8] (Fig. 2.5). In the upper limbs mean arm length is 5–8% less on the affected side. There is a decrease in limb circumference, muscle mass, bone mineral content, and density. The discrepancy in length of one lower limb has a potential to induce secondary changes such as a compensatory forefoot equinus or a pelvic tilt.

Other possible causes for muscle wasting in hemiplegia include

- "end organ resistance" to the hormonal control of growth
- reduced bone mineral density on the affected side from limited weight bearing, worse with severe neurological deficits

Fig. 2.5 Posterior view of the lower limbs during walking illustrating a right hemiplegic gait

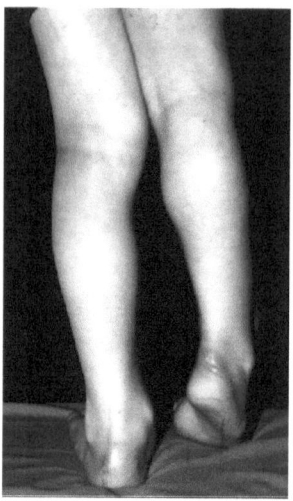

- spasticity reducing sarcomere number and size
- paralysis and disuse atrophy

In diplegia the pelvis is smaller and the lower limbs thinner and shorter than would be expected for the size of the trunk, with the net effect of reduced height and abnormality of posture.

In quadriplegia, growth failure occurs in some 52% [9] The causes are multifactorial and include nutritional contributory factors and bulbar palsy, resulting in generalized and localized growth failure (less than the third centile for height and weight) and markedly reduced muscle glycogen.

In myelomeningocele there is significant dwarfing of the lower limbs and short stature is frequent, especially with higher level lesions. Growth failure results from the neurosegmental motor and sensory level, from the hydrocephalus, from possible renal impairment, and from disordered autonomic control corresponding to the neurological level. Other factors include weight bearing and ambulatory status, vertebral anomalies and curvatures, and, rarely, growth hormone insufficiency.

Other neurological conditions with reduced muscle mass or growth failure include Duchenne dystrophy, Down's syndrome, Prader–Willi syndrome, and Sotos syndrome.

Disuse atrophy can occur very quickly and in one limb may confuse the diagnosis of an osteoid osteoma or other tumor. "Reflex" wasting is secondary to pain from a fracture or synovitis. Muscle wasting may be difficult to evaluate in an obese infant, and imaging (ultrasound or magnetic resonance imaging [MRI]) may be helpful to determine its true extent.

Limb hypertrophy may occur in association with hemihypertrophy of the brain or with the hemangioma of Klippel–Trénaunay syndrome, neurofibromatosis, or hypermelanosis of Ito.

Sensation

Primary sensation can be assessed even in the newborn, particularly with respect to pain. Testing in children is best carried out with a wooden "cocktail stick" or tooth pick rather than the more frightening needle. Dermatome levels are assessed simply in the lower limbs by proceeding anteriorly from the hip to the dorsum of the foot, to the plantar surface of the foot, and then—with the child prone—proceeding up the back of the leg to the buttocks and perianal area. Peripheral nerve lesions can also be identified in this way. The use of cotton wool for light touch and the testing of secondary sensory (proprioceptive) function require significant cooperation from the child and are usually possible only in those of school age or older. The effects of sensory loss are painless fractures, pressure sores and trophic ulcers, and chronic sensory arthropathy (Charcot joints). They are seen in children with myelomeningocele and spinal dysraphic states as well as the congenital sensory neuropathies (Fig. 2.6).

Fig. 2.6 Charcot's joint at the right ankle in a 6-year-old child with hereditary sensory neuropathy characterized by deficiency of small myelinated axons. Marked soft tissue swelling around the ankle joint masks extensive destruction (lytic/sclerotic) changes secondary to chronic trauma to a neuropathic joint

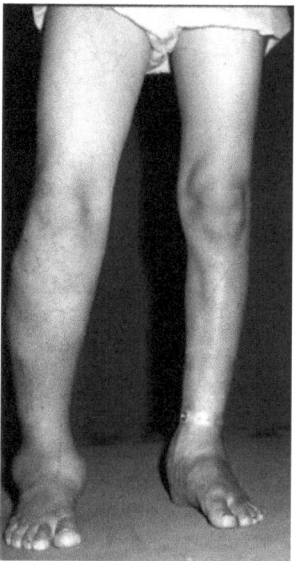

Ataxia

Ataxia means unsteadiness or incoordination and may be induced by cerebellar or spinocerebellar dysfunction, sensory loss, basal ganglia disorders, or spinal cord conditions. In Guillain–Barré syndrome there is a degree of truncal imbalance but no primary ataxia of cerebellar origin, so that all unsteadiness or incoordination is rightly called ataxia, not just that consequent upon cerebellar or spinocerebellar connections.

The development of balance follows a common pattern. While it takes the newborn infant some 12–18 months to be reasonably steady during stance, the newborn animal is steady a short time after birth. The first indication of cerebellar maturation is manifested by "righting reactions," either head-on-trunk righting or trunk-on-pelvis righting, best seen with the child held in a sitting position. These findings are present from 6 or 8 weeks to 3 months. The next level of balance control is seen at 6 months when the sitting child is tilted to either side, extends an arm in a parachute response (lateral parachutes), then an anterior parachute (forward extension of the upper limbs on forward tilting), and finally the posterior parachute at approximately 9 months, when the child extends the arms posteriorly to prevent falling backward. After this stage the child is readily able to change posture and movements independently and with stability. If he can sit and pivot his trunk with stability the primitive reflexes no longer operate and do not require to be tested.

The adult and older child will not use such protective reflexes unless involved in a major fall offsetting any force which attempts to alter the center of gravity and destabilize the trunk by contracting the antigravity muscles to maintain posture. These are dyssynergic movements which are equilibrial reactions and are the most sophisticated evidence of maturation of spinocerebellar connections.

Examination for ataxia is carried out in the upper limbs, trunk and neck, and lower limbs.

Upper Limbs

The finger–nose test is the conventional upper limb test for incoordination, looking for dysmetria and intention tremor (and more accurately disorderly, discontinuous, dysmetric, and off-direction components of the test). It is applicable in older children. As with a lot of paediatric neurology, different testing methods require to be used in order to test the same neurological pathways: for example, the repetitive and sequential finger movements (as standardized by Denckla [10]), rapid hand patting, diadoko- and dysdiadokokinesia, and piano-playing movements. Involuntary movements may be seen in the outstretched hands. Alternatively, in non-compliant younger children functional assessments of coordination can be made during writing, drawing, and coloring.

Truncal Ataxia

In the older child and adolescent this is best assessed with tandem walking where the child walks in a straight line with arms folded on the chest and feet placed heel to toe. Simple gait observation will also give an idea of truncal ataxia, as will standing on either leg or hopping forward, followed by hopping on the spot.

Observation of gait is discussed below but the features of a truncal ataxia are the variability in all gait parameters (speed, direction, step length, double support time, cadence, velocity of swing). The standard deviation of objective measures of these will give an index of ataxia.

Lower Limb Coordination

Many incorrectly think that standing on one leg or hopping is an index of lower limb coordination when in fact it represents truncal control. In the older patient the classical heel–shin test is applied but in the younger child alternative methods of testing are required such as asking the child to jump with both feet together, then both feet apart, and both feet together, repeatedly, and the more difficult jumping with an alternate foot forward. A toe–finger test can be the equivalent of a finger–nose test. The child can be asked to describe the figure 3 or 2 in the air with his big toe. Phasic reflexes in ataxic conditions may be "pendular."

Observational Gait Assessment

Observation of gait is a useful component of the neurological examination, reviewing at least six stride pairs in both the anterior–posterior and lateral direction during each walk. The gait should be at the child's self-selected walking speed. The examiner systematically looks at foot placement and whether this is with a heel–toe disposition with a triple rocker (heel strike, weight bearing, and heel raise/toe-off), flat-footed placement with inversion or eversion, toe-heeling placement, or persistent dynamic equinus. These represent degrees of increasing severity of a typical hemiplegic gait. Foot slapping, a wide base, or other types of foot placement are noted. On the second walk the observer records any change in knee position from extension to 90° of flexion and back again or whether there is any loss of terminal extension prior to heel strike. On the third walk the observer concentrates upon the hip and whether there is any obvious persistent flexion contracture or crouch gait and also whether there is circumduction or waddling. Finally the observer notes any truncal sway.

The important temporal and spatial parameters of gait include the step length, swing time, double support time, cadence (number of steps per minute), walking speed (meters per second), and the velocity of swing phase (See Chapter 6). All of these parameters will change with age and with height. The young child increases his walking speed by increasing cadence whereas the older adolescent increases speed by increasing stride length. Many toddlers have very little double support time. There is a normal asymmetry of gait, the left and right values differing by as much as 10% in any one individual. These asymmetries may relate to established laterality. Wheelwright et al. [11] showed the step length was equal to 43% of the height and that height and gender are major determinants of swing time and cadence, although height, leg length, and gender are independent determinants of double support time.

The normal process of walking involves forward progression of the hip flexors on one side and then heel strike and weight bearing. At this point the individual throws his weight on to the other hip as the other leg achieves heel raise and eventual toe-off. During the swing phase, the leg is similar to a pendulum starting with a zero velocity, increasing to maximum velocity at mid-swing and back to zero velocity at heel strike.

Pattern recognition allows one to distinguish many abnormal gait patterns, for example, the congenital or acquired hemiplegic gait, the diplegic gait, dyskinetic gaits, the gait of Duchenne muscular dystrophy and peripheral neuropathy, the ataxic gait, antalgic gait, festinating gait, and bizarre gaits. The congenital hemiplegic gait pattern (as above), with upper limb flexed and adducted and with flexion at the hip, heel cord and hamstrings, and internal rotation of the lower limb, is different from that of the acquired hemiplegic gait where there is external rotation and abduction in the upper limb and in the foot position. The diplegic gait is essentially a bilateral lower limb hemiplegic-type picture. Dyskinetic gaits show a florid amount of involuntary movements, often with crouch and sway so that it is surprising that upright ambulation is possible. The Duchenne gait is classically with equinus, waddling at the hips, and hyperlordosis. The peripheral neuropathic gait is high stepping and the ataxic gait has variability in all gait parameters as mentioned previously. In practice such children stand on a wide base, make several point turns, do not gauge the slowing down before obstacles, veer off-direction, and progress with variable step lengths and other phases of gait. The antalgic gait is protective against pain. Festinating gaits classical of parkinsonism do not occur in childhood but bizarre gait patterns are seen with psychological disorders, for example, with gross spinal flexion.

Fog Test

For this test the child is asked to walk on the outer borders of both feet and the observer looks for two features:

1. gross asymmetries, the sign of a minimal hemiparesis
2. immature flexion in the upper limbs, a maturation sign

Toe Walking

Toe walking may be normal in the young child who has recently learned to walk. It is often seen in children who are overactive and generally the heel can be brought to the ground in stance. If the habit persists, fixed equinus may develop. Signs of spasticity must be examined for. If a fixed contracture is present, underlying spasticity should be considered a cause although fixed contractures frequently override neurological features as is the case with all positional deformities.

Pes Cavus

In the common equinus deformity this may be at the forefoot or the hind foot (see Chapter 32). In the forefoot variety this may result from persistent toe walking (ballerina syndrome) and develop into a marked cavus foot with claw toes.

The hind foot equinus (Fig. 2.7) may result from paresis (and muscle imbalance), for example, with weak dorsiflexors or a tight calf (tonic spasticity or rigidity), or be consequent upon a short tendon or short leg.

In assessing the foot the Dick or Jack test is often used, passively extending the big toe to see the extent of elevation of the arch of the foot for mobile/structural pes planus. Pes cavus is a feature of diastematomyelia, syringomyelia, spinal intramedullary pathology, such as cysts and progressive conditions, such as Friedreich's ataxia, ataxia telangiectasia, and hereditary motor and sensory neuropathies.

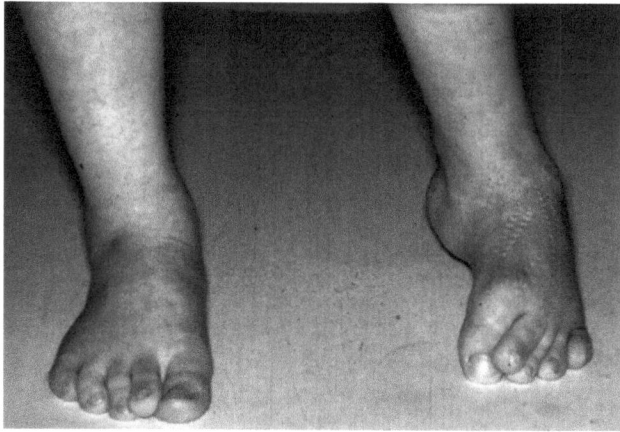

Fig. 2.7 Cavovarus deformity as part of a myelodysplastic limb

Spinal Curvatures

Idiopathic thoracic scoliosis is usually convex to the right; scoliosis to the opposite side is a feature of syringomyelia with Arnold–Chiari malformation (see also Chapter 36).

The spinal curvatures occur with a variety of neurological disorders including diastematomyelia, spinal congenital cysts, Sprengel's shoulder, and the Klippel–Feil deformity. Head tilt may be a manifestation of cerebellar hemisphere tumor before the classical cerebellar signs or signs of raised intracranial pressure occur.

The purpose of developmental screening and testing is to screen for pathology, relying upon a combination of reported developmental milestones and clinical examination. Such motor delay triggers a need for investigations such as creatinine phosphokinase levels, neurophysiology, and imaging, which clarify the diagnosis. The delay in neurodevelopmental acquisition of posture and movement milestones is noted. A fuller developmental assessment (e.g., Griffiths, test) will depict other aspects of development and will provide an indication of the effect that the motor disorder has had on other areas of the child's development. Following appropriate treatment or therapy a reassessment of the neurodevelopmental status will monitor the benefits of treatments.

Diseases Which Require Special Neurodevelopmental Examination of the Motor System

Neural Tube Defects

Newborn babies with myelomeningocele (see Chapter 17) require a detailed examination of the lower limbs shortly after birth in order to derive the neurosegmental motor sensory and reflex levels. Examination will also identify the features of the "isolated cord" which are

- isolated muscle spasticity
- loss of reciprocal inhibition
- reflexes elicited in toes, hamstrings, and tibialis anterior
- flexor withdrawal with oscillation
- no extensor activity
- flexor pattern of tone if long segment
- anal reflex preservation
- dermatome to myotome responses
- spastic pelvic floor and bladder neck
- deformity due to unopposed spastic muscles
- wide afferent field with crossed adductor responses
- spontaneous spinal myoclonus

In addition to these observations, detailed clinical examination of power, reflexes, sensation, and deformity is recorded at the ankle, foot, knee, hip, and spine.

The pattern of cord involvement can be deduced, such as the type 1 cord in which the myelomeningocele destroys the cord terminally to a variable height causing flaccidity, areflexia, and anesthesia in the distal segment. The lowest normally functioning neurosegmental level describes the lesion level. The neurological level is the functionally important level, not the lesion level or vertebral level.

In type 2 cord involvement, the myelomeningocele destroys a more proximal area of the spinal cord to a variable degree, leaving normal but isolated cord distally. The isolated cord here may be a short segment or a long segment which is akin to a transverse myelitic lesion.

Type 3 is where the myelomeningocele only partially destroys the cord, for example, in the thoracolumbar region, and some descending long tracks will be preserved and others halted at the upper level of the lesion. Only examination of the lower limbs will decide which are intact.

Type 4 is an incomplete conus lesion where the terminal part of the cord is incompletely involved and again some descending tracts descend the full length of the cord whereas others do not.

From a deformity point of view, the pattern of cord involvement is very important. In type 1 normal power muscle groups oppose flaccid muscle groups across joints; in type 2 flaccid muscle opposes spastic muscle groups. The mechanism of deformity in children with neural tube defects is due to

- an imbalance of muscle action across joints
- positional deformity either in utero or acquired postnatally

Examination of these infants involves ultrasound of the hips, bladder, and kidneys; ultrasound or MRI scanning of the spinal cord and spine; as well as imaging of the Chiari 2 malformation and hydrocephalus. The neurosegmental motor levels are particularly important for predicting subsequent walking, and children with MRC 3 power or better in the quadriceps (L3, 4) are generally ambulant with below-knee orthoses or aids. Children with higher motor levels require above-knee bracing and sticks or hip guidance or reciprocating gait orthoses. Hip dislocation is not a separate congenital malformation but a result of muscle imbalance occurring early in high-level and low-level lesions but not in mid-lumbar level lesions.

Chiari Malformation

The Chiari 1 malformation occurs where there is descent of the cerebellar tonsils through the foramen magnum. The Chiari 2 malformation occurs in association with myelomeningocele and the descent of the tonsils and vermis. The Chiari 3 malformation is an occipital or cervical meningocele with enclosed cerebral tissue and the Chiari 4 malformation is cerebellar hypoplasia.

It is of theoretical importance whether the descending tissue is the cerebellar tonsils or vermis, and on MRI a descent of 2 cm below the foramen magnum is considered significant. The appearance of descending cerebellar tissue is important and, if rounded, probably indicates that there is no significant impaction. The sharply contoured descending portion is more indicative of tightness at the craniocervical junction. T2 MRI images may exaggerate the amount of surrounding subarachnoid space available.

All children with spina bifida should be routinely checked for signs of impaction or cavitation (hydromyelia or syringomyelia) in the cervical cord as a result of Chiari malformation. They should be checked for muscle power distally in the upper limbs and be examined for wasting of the thenar/hypothenar muscle groups and fasciculation in the hands or shoulders. Reflexes (biceps and triceps) are tested and impaired bulbar function checked (difficulty with swallowing and speech or "strain"-type headaches on coughing or sneezing).

Brisk upper limb reflexes alone will indicate a degree of impaction, and cavitation will produce signs of lower motor neurone lesion in the upper limbs. Somatosensory potentials (although technically difficult to obtain in the infant and young child) from the upper limbs along with sequential imaging and clinical examination will help to decide whether occipital and cervical decompression are indicated.

Tethered Cord

The normal spinal conus terminates at L1 but may be considerably lower if tethered to a fatty lump (lipomeningocele) or paired myelomeningocele. Tethering of the cord or filum may occur at various levels and the child presents with a loss of acquired function which may be motor, sensory, or reflex, a change in bladder innervation, or pain in the back or lower limbs. Examination of the lower limbs will confirm a changed neurosegmental level (there may be a pre-existing myelodysplasia) and somatosensory evoked potentials from the lower limbs likewise show a changed pattern. Clinical and physiological changes will differentiate a radiological tethering from symptomatic tethering of the cord. The child may become symptomatic during periods of rapid linear growth; height is routinely measured at all outpatient visits. Spinal dysraphic states are suspected if there is a vascular pigmented nevus, hairy patch, pit, or lipoma near the distal midline of the spine.

Classically the myelodysplastic leg is thin with cavovarus deformity and autonomic (trophic) changes. With only one leg involved the child cannot develop a neuropathic bladder.

Duchenne and Other Muscular Dystrophies

Clinically muscular dystrophy is suspected because of a delay in the motor milestones of a young boy with calf hypertrophy and a positive Gower's sign. Ankle reflexes may be lost and the child walks on his toes with a waddling gait and a severe lordosis.

The clinical progress of Duchenne dystrophy may be monitored by following a scale to monitor the rate of progression of this regressive condition [12]:

1. walks and climbs stairs without assistance
2. walks and climbs stairs with aid of railing
3. walks and climbs stairs slowly with aid of railing (>25 s for eight standard steps)
4. walks unassisted and rises from chair but cannot climb stairs
5. walks unassisted but cannot rise from chair or climb stairs
6. walks only with assistance or walks independently with long leg braces
7. walks in leg braces but requires assistance for balance
8. stands in long leg braces but unable to walk even with assistance
9. remains in wheelchair or bed

Clinical slowing of progression is achieved by maintaining ambulation, by corrective scoliosis surgery, and by nocturnal continuous positive airways pressure (CPAP) ventilation. Cyclical steroids are also tried. This is further discussed in Chapter 16.

Congenital Motor Disorders (Cerebral Palsy)

Congenital motor disorders (cerebral palsy) are discussed in Chapter 19, but here are detailed: (1) the range of neurological abnormalities in a hemiplegia, (2) "cerebral palsy in evolution," (3) transient dystonia of prematurity, and (4) "minimal hemiplegia."

Components of Hemiplegia

Although a hemiplegia appears to be a homogeneous entity, it consists of a number of different components including dyspraxia, peripheral weakness, impaired proximal fly-swatting movements, spasticity/rigidity, brisk tendon reflexes, extensor plantar responses, abnormal limb posture, asymmetrical protective reflexes, involuntary movements (athetoid postures), abnormal sensation, vasomotor changes, unilateral primitive reflexes, retention of grasp reflex, excessive "associated" and "mirror" movements, and abnormal growth.

Recognition of cerebral palsy in evolution can be challenging for the neurologist. In early infancy hemiplegic signs may not be obvious and may take 6–9 months to evolve. A hint to the future motor pattern may be seen with asymmetry of the phasic reflexes, preference for voluntary movement on one side, asymmetrical parachute responses or delay in sitting, kicking one leg more than the other, and developing a strong hand preference in infancy.

Transient Dystonia Following Prematurity

This is often seen in mid-infancy with a prone/supine discrepancy, the child arching his back and extending the limbs when held vertical or placed prone and adopting a more flexor pattern when in supine. The transient rigidity picture is to be distinguished from the more florid evolution of dystonic or spastic diplegia or quadriplegia. It is said that cerebral palsy occurs during the phase of brain growth, in the first 4 years of life, but can be diagnosed when the motor features are present before this, for example, in dyskinetic cerebral palsy.

Minimal Hemiplegia

A minimal hemiplegia can be distinguished clinically only with difficulty by assessing distal fine finger movements (Denckla test [10]) or fastening buttons, a mild pronator catch, asymmetrical or associated movements on fog testing, mild weakness of grasp, failure to swing the arm during walking, or exaggerated asymmetry of nail breadths.

Hereditary Sensory Motor Neuropathies

There are a number of clinically and genetically distinct orders in which abnormalities of sensory motor nerves are prominent. They have to be distinguished from conditions in which peripheral neuropathy is part of a more generalized neuraxial abnormality such as Friedrich's ataxia or motor chromatic leukodystrophy, and from sensory neuropathies in which the motor nerves are spared but may produce neuropathic joints, fractures, and ulceration. Of the six types, the most important to the orthopaedic surgeon is type 1 Charcot–Marie–Tooth disease, an autosomal dominant disorder often presenting with pes cavus, equinus, and broadening of the forefoot. Kyphosis and scoliosis may present later. Tendon jerks are lost early and sensory impairment (joint position and vibration) may develop. The "champagne bottle" leg deformity is rarely seen in children. In this condition examination of the parents may be helpful.

Among sporadic cases 30% are new, dominant mutations and the remainder recessive. A few have gender-linked recessive inheritance. In type 2, axonal neuropathy is more slowly progressive and sensory impairment less obvious. Type 3 is more severe, with club feet, severe muscle wasting and weakness, and impairment of all sensory modalities. There is also proximal involvement with hip dislocation, and scoliosis is seen eventually. In this type there is hypertrophic interstitial neuropathy with onion skin formation seen microscopically and palpable thickening of subcutaneous nerves. Such patients do not tolerate prolonged immobilization, for example, after corrective surgery. Genetic counseling can be very helpful.

The Profoundly Handicapped Child

The neuromotor patterns of the profoundly handicapped child are illustrated in Fig. 2.8, and such children are prone to secondary positional deformity (wind sweeping deformity) where, for example, in side lying, the plane of the shoulder and hip is not aligned. The child corkscrews about a longitudinal access giving rise to scoliosis, pelvic obliquity, leg length discrepancy, plagiocephaly, bat ear, thoracic asymmetry, and a skew posture of the lower limbs. The deformation overrides the original neurological pattern. This is the most severe type of positional deformity and results from the effects of gravity upon a child who is unable to change position. Positional deformity may occur in normal infants, for example, following prematurity with the squint baby or molded baby syndrome. At 3 months of age assessment of positional asymmetries is at its most difficult, particularly in deciding whether there is an underlying neuromotor condition predisposing to it.

Children recovering from serious traumatic brain injury or meningitis are especially prone to developing positional deformities superimposed upon residual neurological deficits. Their care demands scrupulous attention to postural turning and nursing principles.

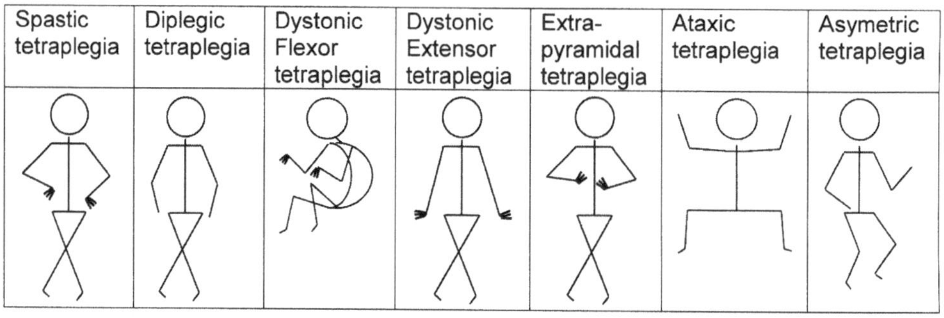

Fig. 2.8 Schematic of the
different tetraplegic motor
patterns seen in the profoundly
handicapped child

Spastic tetraplegia	Diplegic tetraplegia	Dystonic Flexor tetraplegia	Dystonic Extensor tetraplegia	Extra-pyramidal tetraplegia	Ataxic tetraplegia	Asymetric tetraplegia

References

1. Minns RA, Sobkowiak CA, Skardoutsou A, et al. Upper limb function in Spina Bifida. Zeitschrift fur Kinderchirurgie 1977; 22:(4):493–506.

2. Yakovlev PI, Lecours A-R. The myelogenetic cycles of regional maturation of the brain. In: Minkowski A, ed. Regional Development of the Brain in Early Life. Oxford: Blackwell; 1967:3–70.

3. Medical Research Council. Aids to the investigation of peripheral nerve injuries. War Memorandum No 7 ed. London: HMSO, 1943.

4. Holmes G. The Croonian lectures on the clinical symptoms of cerebellar disease. Lancet 1922; 199:(5155):1177–1182.

5. American Academy of Orthopaedic Surgeons. Joint Motion. Method of measuring and recording. Edinburgh: Churchill Livingston, 1965.

6. Ashworth B. Preliminary trial of carisoprodol in multiple sclerosis. Practitioner 1964; 192:540–542.

7. Aram DM, Ekelman BL, Satz P. Trophic changes following early unilateral injury to the brain. Dev Med Child Neurol 1986; 28:(2):165–170.

8. Lin JP, Brown JK. Peripheral and central mechanisms of hindfoot equinus in childhood hemiplegia. Dev Med Child Neurol 1992; 34:(11):949–965.

9. Minns RA, Wong B, Brown JK, Fraser WI. Neuro-developmental study of profoundly mentally handicapped children in hospital care. J Ment Defic Res 1989; 33:(Pt 6):439–454.

10. Denckla MB. Development of speed in repetitive and successive finger-movements in normal children. Dev Med Child Neurol 1973; 15:(5):635–645.

11. Wheelwright EF, Minns RA, Elton RA, Law HT. Temporal and spatial parameters of gait in children. II: Pathological gait. Dev Med Child Neurol 1993; 35:(2):114–125.

12. Vignos PJ. Rehabilitation in the myopathies. In: Vinken PJ, Bruyn GW, eds. Handbook of Clinical Neurology. Amsterdam: North-Holland Pub. Co.; 1979.

Chapter 3

Hereditary and Developmental Neuromuscular Disorders

Eugene E. Bleck and James E. Robb

Introduction

This chapter considers those conditions characterized by weakness resulting from pathology primarily in the muscles or the anterior horn cells of the spinal cord. In their later stages these disorders have recognizable clinical features, but in the early stages all share a common set of symptoms and physical signs. Generally, motor disorders are either genetic or acquired. Children with the former tend to present with weakness and delayed motor skills whereas those with the acquired type usually have fairly rapid progression of weakness and loss of function. Children who are floppy at birth are likely to be evaluated initially by a paediatrician or paediatric neurologist but the orthopaedic surgeon may be the first specialist to assess a child with a walking difficulty caused by Duchenne's or Becker's dystrophy.

Assessment

Symptoms

The majority of children with a muscle disorder will present with delayed motor milestones. An experienced mother may recognize that her child has moved less than usual in utero. The history should confirm developmental milestones and, if the motor problem was not noticed in early development, at what age the deterioration in motor development occurred. After birth the affected child may be weak and floppy (Fig. 3.1) and unlike other children may present with delayed sitting, crawling, or walking. However, this is also seen in children with global developmental delay. Normally, a term infant will sit at 6 months, crawl at 9 months, stand at 10 months, and walk at 12–14 months. About 10% of

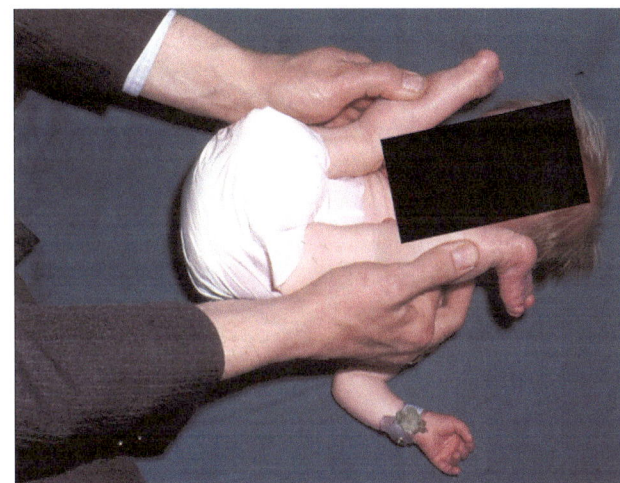

Fig. 3.1 Floppy baby. Courtesy of Dr P. Eunson

children bottom-shuffle rather than crawl, and 97% walk six steps unaided by 18 months.

The most common symptoms that cause parents to seek consultation are listed in Table 3.1. It is salutary to remember that Read and Galasko [1] reported a mean delay of 2 years in making the diagnosis of Duchenne muscular dystrophy (DMD), particularly on the part of orthopaedic surgeons.

Examination

A standard orthopaedic examination including a neurological assessment is required but will also focus on delayed motor milestones, muscle strength and tone, muscle fasciculation, and gait. Some conditions are associated with learning difficulties, for example, DMD. Sensation will be normal in muscular dystrophies, spinal muscular atrophy (SMA), myopathy, and myasthenia gravis but impaired in sensorimotor neuropathies such as Charcot–Marie–Tooth disease.

The presence of joint contractures at birth should alert the clinician to the possibility of arthrogryposis (Fig. 3.2)

E.E. Bleck (✉)
Department of Orthopaedic Surgery, Stanford University School of Medicine, Stanford, CA, USA

Table 3.1 Common symptoms of neuromuscular disease

Infancy	Floppy baby
	Slow development; not sitting unaided at 9 months
	Muscles lack consistency and tone
Childhood	Tiptoeing (most common complaint in Duchenne muscular dystrophy)
	Clumsy; awkward
	Cannot keep up with other children
	Runs strangely
	Seems weak and fatigues easily
	Waddling gait
	Posture is poor; stands with "sway-back and pot-belly"
	Cannot cut with scissors in kindergarten
	Printing by hand or writing is slow and labored
	Is he/she "learning disabled?"

impairment. In some conditions, both central and peripheral hypotonia may coexist [2].

Posture

Slight degrees of shift of the spine from the midline may be noted in addition to a loin crease, both of which are early signs of scoliosis which can be an early manifestation of neuromuscular disease. Forward drooping of the shoulders, a prominent abdomen, or lumbar lordosis should arouse suspicion (Fig. 3.3). Winging of the scapula can be mistaken for a benign, slumped posture.

In the young infant a hypotonic posture may be noted (Fig. 3.4) and head lag seen when pulling the infant from supine to sitting (Fig. 3.5). "Slip through" at the shoulder girdle may occur when the infant is held vertically under

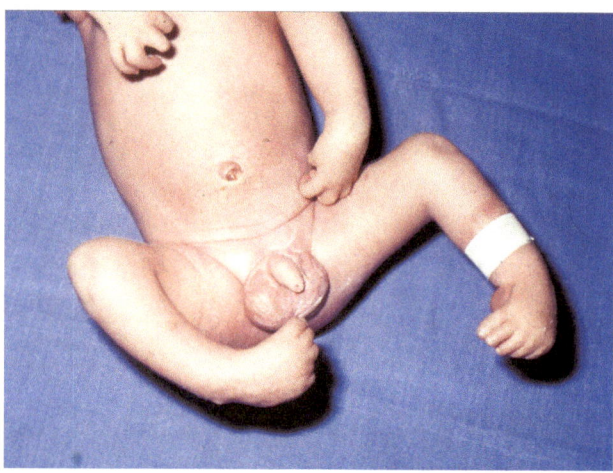

Fig. 3.2 Arthrogryposis. Courtesy of Dr P. Eunson

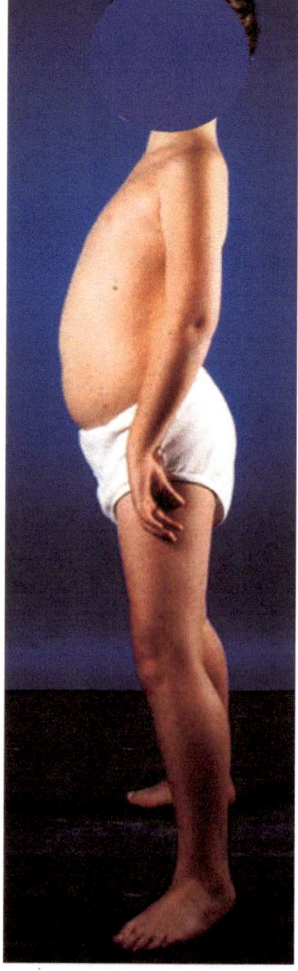

Fig. 3.3 Prominent abdomen and lumbar lordosis in DMD. Note the pseudo-hypertrophy of the calves

as well as neuromuscular disorders that are associated with low tone, muscle imbalance, or paralysis. This should be distinguished from "packaging disorders."

It may also be useful to determine if the infant has a central or peripheral type of hypotonia. Paralytic hypotonia with significant weakness suggests a peripheral neuromuscular problem such as SMA, neuropathy, myopathy, muscle dystrophies, or myasthenic syndromes. A non-paralytic hypotonia without significant weakness suggests a central cause, which may be neurological, genetic, syndromic, or metabolic. A peripheral problem may be associated with a delay in motor milestones but relatively normal social and cognitive development whereas a central problem may be associated with motor delay and social and cognitive

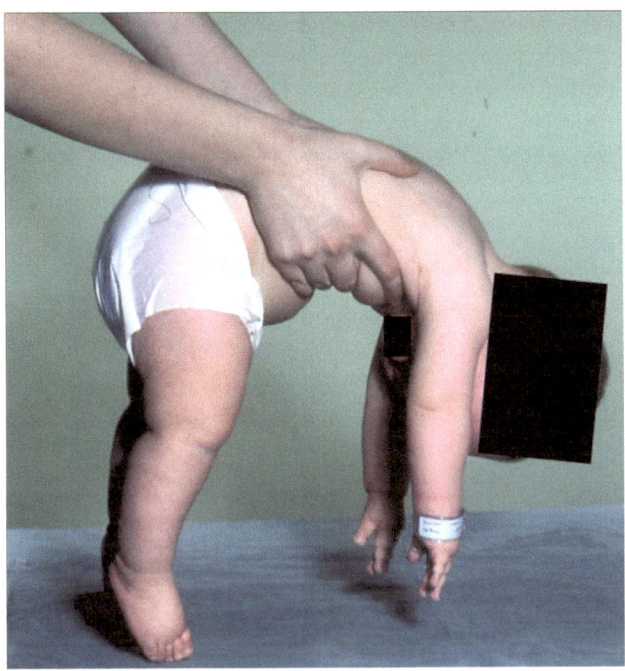

Fig. 3.4 Hypotonic posture. Courtesy of Dr P. Eunson

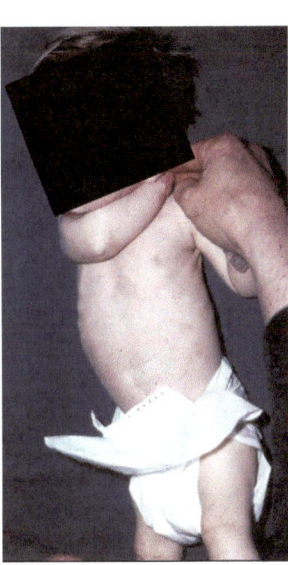

Fig. 3.6 Scarf sign. Illustration courtesy of Dr P. Eunson

Muscular Testing and Observation

Activity Test

The child should be asked to walk on his heels, sit on the floor and then rise, stand on one foot, hop, step up and down from a stool, climb stairs, and walk on tiptoe. Gower's sign is when the child has to use the hands and arms to "walk" up the body from a squatting position due to lack of lower extremity muscle strength (Fig. 3.7). One-sided tiptoeing, while the examiner holds the child's hand for balance, is a useful way of demonstrating significant gastrocnemius–soleus weakness. Normally, a child should be able to rise on one foot 8–9 times in sequence. Trendelenburg sign may be difficult to elicit in a normal child younger than 6 or 7 years because of a lack of fully developed balance reactions.

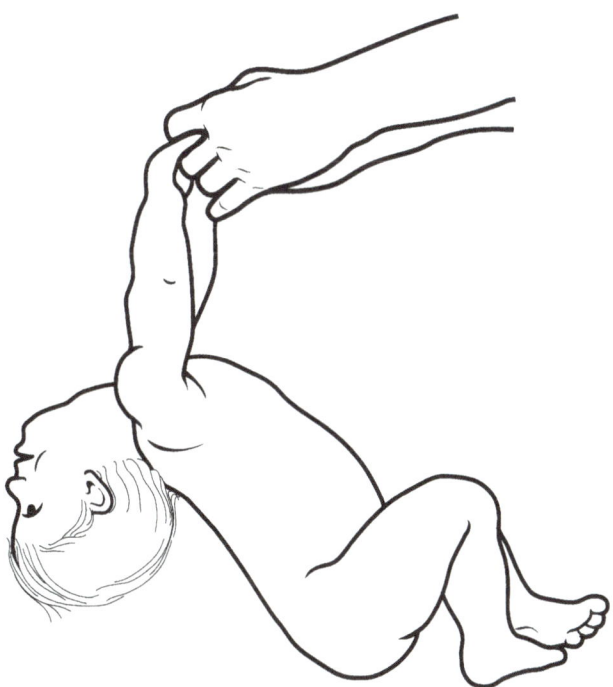

Fig. 3.5 Head lag

the arms and the "scarf sign" also indicates shoulder girdle weakness (Fig. 3.6). The infant may not be able to bear weight through the legs when supported under the axillae. In older infants the ability to roll over, sit unaided, and to pull to stand should be noted.

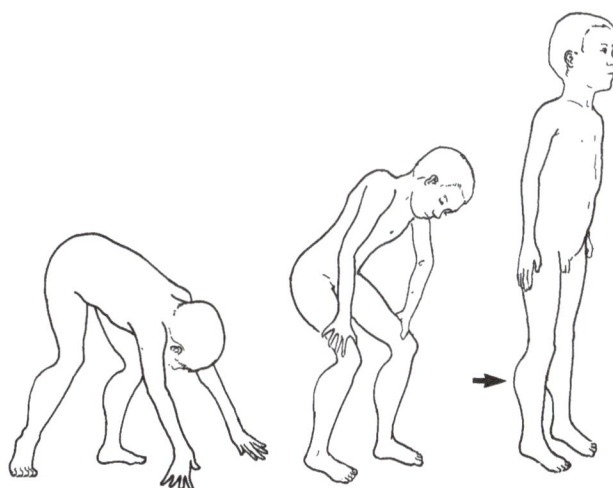

Fig. 3.7 Gower's sign

Manual Muscle Testing

Manual muscle testing can be difficult in younger children but in those who can cooperate manual muscle testing and Medical Research Council (MRC) grading should be performed (Table 3.2).

Table 3.2 Manual muscle testing (MRC grading)

Power 5 (normal)	The portion of the limb being tested moves through its full range against gravity and maximum resistance
Power 4 (good)	Moves against gravity and moderate resistance
Power 3 (fair)	Moves against gravity but not against resistance
Power 2 (poor)	Moves only with gravity eliminated
Power 1 (trace)	Flicker of contraction only
Power 0 (zero)	No movement

Muscle Tone

Although contemporary physiotherapists commonly use the term "tone," its meaning is poorly defined. The French use the terms *extensibilité*—the amount of lengthening permitted by the muscle—and "passivité"—denoting the lack of resistance to passive movement [3]. *Passivité* can be assessed by grasping the child's forearm and flapping the wrist up and down rapidly. The real value of the term is in the diagnosis of the "floppy" or hypotonic infant [4]; later in childhood, the sign is less useful. The presence of contractures at birth suggests a peripheral neuromuscular disorder such as congenital muscular dystrophy and may also be seen in any disorder that limits fetal movement such as spina bifida.

Atrophy and Hypertrophy

The degree of atrophy in lower motor neurone disease generally correlates with the amount of weakness, whereas in primary myopathies it does not. Hypertrophy is most noticeable in myotonia congenita, in which muscle strength is proportional to bulk. Early in DMD the calf, deltoid, and vastus lateralis muscles will appear hypertrophied. In later stages "pseudohypertrophy" occurs as the muscle fibers are replaced by fat (Fig. 3.3). Three myopathies are characterized by severe weakness but no atrophy: myasthenia gravis, polymyositis, and periodic paralysis. This observation is very important because these three myopathies are among the few that can be treated.

Fasciculations

Spontaneous twitching of the muscles, especially in the calf, the intrinsic muscles of the hand, and the tongue, characterizes a degenerating anterior horn cell disease. Even if fasciculations are not seen, anterior horn cell disease cannot be ruled out, as denervation fibrillation (arrhythmic "blips" that can be seen only on the electromyograph [EMG]) may still be present.

Reflexes

The deep tendon reflexes usually disappear early in the neuropathies and diminish in parallel with increasing muscle weakness in the myopathies. They are preserved in polymyositis and myasthenia gravis. The plantar responses are always flexor (negative Babinski sign) in the myopathies and neuropathies except in the rare case of spinal muscular atrophy with pyramidal tract involvement [5]. If extensor responses occur, an upper motor neurone disorder should be suspected.

Gait

Older children should be asked to walk, if possible, along a well-lit walkway or corridor and their gait observed to allow assessment of the stance and swing phases in the sagittal plane and rotation in the transverse plane (see Chapter 6). A waddling gait may not necessarily represent hip abductor weakness and hip dysplasia should be excluded radiologically. A high-stepping gait is associated with weakness of ankle dorsiflexion and a toe-drag gait with spasticity. When asked to run, a child with barely perceptible spastic hemiplegia will often flex the elbow and clench the fist on the involved side so attention should be paid to the upper limbs when observing a gait. A child with muscle weakness appears labored when running and may mimic ataxia. Three-dimensional gait analysis is useful in providing a baseline evaluation of gait for future reference.

Laboratory Investigations

Serum Enzymes

By far the most sensitive test in the diagnosis of DMD is the measurement of serum creatine kinase (CK). Very high levels occur before the onset of symptoms and signs and gradually decrease as the disease progresses because the muscle is replaced by fat. The concentration of serum aldolase is also elevated in DMD. Serum lactate and pyruvate should be obtained if a mitochondrial disease is suspected. If congenital hypothyroidism is suspected the infant should have the thyroid function checked. An edrophonium test is used to diagnose myasthenia gravis.

Electromyography

DNA testing is supplanting EMG studies in the diagnosis of muscle disorders and is used to support the diagnosis of a muscle disease. EMG features in peripheral hypotonia are shown in Table 3.3.

Table 3.3 EMG features in peripheral hypotonia

Neurogenic	Large amplitude action potentials, reduced interference pattern, increased internal instability
Myopathic	Small amplitude action potentials with increased interference pattern
Myotonic	Increased insertional activity
Myasthenic	Abnormal repetitive and single fiber studies

Adapted from Gowda et al. [2]

Muscle Biopsy

The surgeon should consult with the pathologist before undertaking a muscle biopsy to ensure that the specimen will be of adequate size, transported in the correct medium, and delivered at an appropriate time of day to allow processing. The surgeon should also check with the pathologist whether a core needle biopsy would suffice or whether an open biopsy is preferred. The muscle chosen for biopsy should be abnormal and a pre-biopsy magnetic resonance image (MRI) may help to identify areas of abnormality if there is doubt. Biopsies are usually obtained from the vastus lateralis or deltoid, as they are proximal and often affected early in myopathies and dystrophies. Generally, the labeled biopsy specimen is placed on a damp saline swab and needs to be sent fresh to the laboratory promptly to avoid desiccation. Examples of normal muscle and that seen in DMD are illustrated in Fig. 3.8.

Etiology and Inheritance

Most muscle disorders, except polymyositis, have defined patterns of inheritance: the dystrophies and myopathies are usually autosomal dominant or sex-linked, whereas the atrophies are generally autosomal recessive. A positive family history is not invariable, as spontaneous mutations may occur. The responsible gene in Duchenne and Becker muscular dystrophies has been identified on the xp21 region of the X-chromosome, and the genetic locus for SMA has been identified on chromosome 5q. Advances in genetic research offer the prospect of gene therapies for genetically determined muscle disease and now that the first trials of gene therapy for DMD are starting it is important to know the exact mutation for each boy. Families can also be counseled appropriately about the risk of future children being affected by a genetically based disorder.

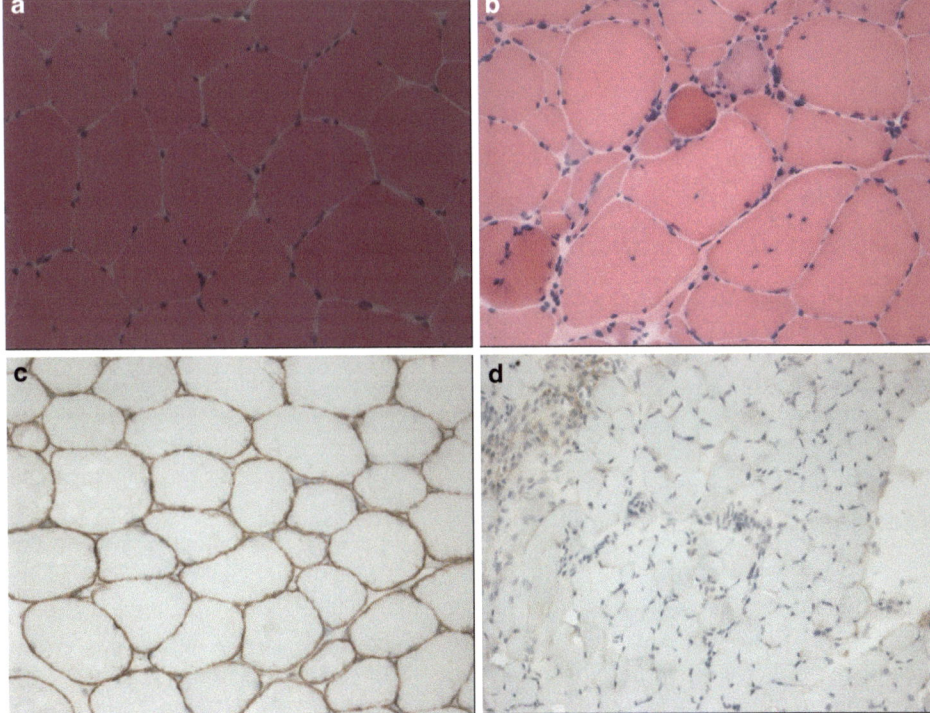

Fig. 3.8 (**a**) Normal muscle (H&E stain ×20 magnification). (**b**) Duchenne muscle showing fiber splitting and hypercontracted (red) fibers (H&E stain ×40 magnification). (**c**) Immunohistochemistry for dystrophin in normal muscle (×40 magnification). (**d**) Immunohistochemistry for dystrophin which is absent in Duchenne muscle (×40 magnification). Illustrations courtesy of Dr C. Smith

Differential Diagnosis

Figure 3.9 categorizes anatomically the most common neuromuscular disorders that need to be considered in children, showing the relevant clinical, hereditary, and laboratory details.

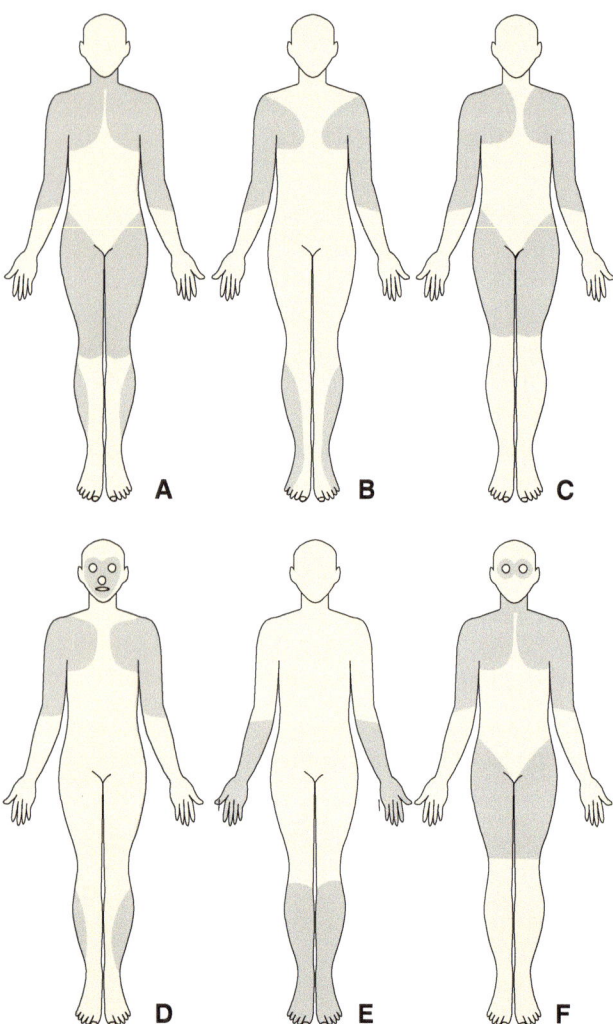

Fig. 3.9 General distribution of the muscle dystrophies (**a**) Duchenne and Becker. (**b**) Emery–Dreyfuss. (**c**) Limb-girdle. (**d**) Fascio-scapulo-humeral. (**e**) Distal. (**f**) Occulopharyngeal. *Shaded* = affected areas. After Emery AE [16]

Management

The child is best managed through a neuromuscular clinic offering care from a range of disciplines, typically paediatric neurology, orthopaedics, cardiology, respiratory medicine, physiotherapy, occupational and speech therapy, orthotic provision, and rehabilitation technology. The aims of management are summarized below (see also Chapter 3).

Physiotherapy and Occupational Therapy

The emphasis is upon mobility and independence. The child should be moved out of the seated position during the day and allowed to roll about and play on a mat. This may be more effective than passive stretching although every attempt should be made to counteract the remorseless development of contractures and the effects of gravity. Walking should be encouraged, but eventually proves impossible when the hip abductor and extensor muscles weaken to MRC grade III or less. Adaptive physiotherapy and wheelchair games seem to encourage respiratory exchange and avoid repetitive and tedious exercises. Standing frames are useful to give a child a different perception of the environment from that seen from a wheelchair and can also provide a passive stretch to joints of the lower limb. Swimming in a heated pool is ideal, as water allows the trunk and limbs to move as freely as possible and at the same time provides resistance to maintain muscle strength.

External supports should be used to maintain walking ability and transfer skills. When this is no longer possible, the child should be provided with a manual or powered wheelchair as appropriate.

Physiotherapy is also required for those children with respiratory impairment to maintain for as long as possible the child's ability to clear secretions and maintain an adequate tidal volume.

Aids to daily living and modification of the child's environment should include ground floor accommodation, bathroom alterations, and provision of a hoisting system. Powered wheelchairs that allow the patient to recline, sit up, and stand up are available. Electrically operated beds afford comfort when resting and sleeping. Electric toothbrushes and bath aids, alteration in shower cubicle entrances, and bidets that attach to toilet seats to obviate the need for laborious and often impossible paper cleansing have improved independence as well as eased the constant burden on the family and carers. Electronic environmental controls with sensitive pressure switches put the command of much of the household at the fingertips and can be used for communication devices. Patients with impaired breathing can be assisted by ventilatory systems powered from their wheelchair's batteries. Transport in adapted cars or vans has expanded the horizon of these children and increased the freedom of the family. Wheelchair-accessible residences, public buildings, streets, and pavements should provide freedom of movement and improved social contact.

Orthotics

Ankle–foot orthoses (AFOs) are useful in preventing equinus contracture, providing stability in stance and accommodating a foot or ankle deformity. AFOs are useful as long as the child has the hip muscle power to walk. Bracing at the knee, hip, and trunk is too cumbersome to permit efficient walking and knee–ankle–foot orthoses (KAFOs) and hip–knee–ankle–foot orthoses (HKAFOs) are not recommended. Orthoses do not prevent hip flexion contractures because the patient merely develops a greater compensatory lumbar lordosis. Hip flexion contractures greater than 45° lead to loss of standing ability.

Thoraco-lumbar-sacral orthoses (TLSOs) are ineffective in preventing the progression of a neuromuscular scoliosis and there may also be concerns that the orthosis will restrict chest wall expansion in a child who already suffers respiratory compromise. The Milwaukee brace, a cervical-thoracic-lumbar-sacral orthosis, is also contraindicated for the same reason and extensive bracing can interfere with comfortable sitting in a wheelchair. However, a TLSO may be used to stabilize the trunk to free the arms so the child can operate an electric wheelchair or eat, for example. The TLSO may also "hold" a scoliosis until the child is old enough to undergo spinal instrumentation and fusion [6]. Molded seating may be necessary to accommodate a scoliosis in those children for whom spinal surgery is contraindicated.

Cardiopulmonary Function

Cardiomyopathy occurs in muscle disorders, such as Becker muscular dystrophy (BMD) and in disorders of glycogen and lipid use. Screening and review by a paediatric cardiologist is desirable and also necessary before consideration of extensive surgery such as spinal stabilization and fusion.

Diaphragmatic and intercostal muscle weakness results in diminished respiratory function. It usually occurs insidiously and sleep apnea may be the first presenting sign; sleep studies are then required. As respiratory function deteriorates the child has difficulty in clearing secretions, which may also be compounded by a bulbar palsy resulting in an unsafe swallow and aspiration pneumonia.

Non-invasive mechanical ventilation can be considered in the later stages of deteriorating pulmonary function. Bi-level positive airway pressure may be helpful for sleep apnea. The decision to proceed to tracheostomy and formal ventilation is a difficult one in the face of incurable, progressive muscle disease and is a quandary for the child, parents, and carers.

Prevention of Infection and Nutrition

Children with impaired respiratory function are at risk of chest infection so an annual influenza vaccination and pneumococcus immunization are recommended. Adequate nutrition is required to ensure growth and short-term nasogastric feeding may be necessary in the acute stages of an infective illness to minimize catabolism. A bulbar palsy may necessitate percutaneous enteral feeding. For some children gastro-esophageal reflux is an associated problem that can be helped by endoscopic fundoplication. Surgery, if required, is best performed at an early stage because of the associated cardiopulmonary compromise.

Orthopaedic Surgery

Scoliosis occurs in 90% of the spinal muscular atrophies, DMD, and some of the myopathies. Fortunately, in the past 20 years the development of spinal instrumentation has allowed surgical correction before respiratory compromise becomes too great and the operative risk untenable. Transdiaphragmatic approaches to the spine for disc excision should be avoided in children with impaired cardiorespiratory function. The use of cell-saver devices and donor bone graft is widespread in these extensive spinal fusions. Although spinal fusion is generally successful in improving comfort for seating, patients and parents should be aware that the improved spinal alignment may impair the ability of the child to feed independently. When there is upper limb weakness, the loss of the ability to bring the mouth toward the hand when the spine was collapsed pre-operatively can be lost post-operatively.

Flexion contractures of the hip and knee and equinus and varus of the ankle and foot are common in neuromuscular disorders and are inevitable in the non-walking child whose limb alignment adapts to the shape of their wheelchair. Muscle and tendon lengthenings at the hip and knee in the non-walker are not generally effective. However, management of equinus of the ankle and varus of the foot are exceptions to this limited surgical perspective as equinovarus impairs proper foot contact with the child's immediate environment. This foot posture may produce areas of high contact pressure on the lateral border of the foot and/or toes, cause difficulty in shoe wear fitting and/or orthoses, and preclude a comfortable resting position of the foot on the footplate of a wheelchair for the non-walker.

Hip subluxation and dislocation occur frequently in the myopathies and may account for the failure to maintain reduction in some cases of presumed developmental dysplasia of the hip. The diagnosis of a myopathy should alert the surgeon and the family to a guarded prognosis and the likely development of contractures despite physiotherapy [7].

Spinal Muscular Atrophy

The incidence of SMA is approximately 1 in 15,000 to 1 in 20,000 live births [8]. All forms of SMA involve selective destruction of anterior horn cells and all patients have muscle weakness.

Classification and Clinical Features

SMA is a heterogeneous condition but for clinical purposes can be classified into three types according to the patient's age at the onset of the disease.

Type I—Acute Infantile (Werdnig–Hoffmann's) Disease

The onset of this form is from birth to 6 months and the infant presents with floppy limbs and trunk and paucity of limb movement. Affected infants appear alert and the facial muscles are initially spared. Weakness is progressive and infants experience swallowing and breathing difficulties. As the weakness progresses the upper and lower limbs may be positioned in the "pithed frog" posture with abduction and external rotation at the hips and shoulders. The mean survival is 6 months and 95% of affected infants are dead by 18 months. The use of long-term ventilation in severe SMA is controversial.

Type II—Chronic Infantile (Intermediate Group)

The chronic infantile form of spinal muscular atrophy has an onset from 6 months of age and usually manifests by the age of 2 years, after which it is slowly progressive. The infant usually attains head control and the majority of children achieve sitting balance but not independent walking. Life expectancy can extend into the third decade of life. Progressive scoliosis, limb contractures, and diminished vital capacity are the rule.

Type III—Chronic Proximal (Kugelberg–Welander)

Type III is usually diagnosed in later childhood between the ages of 2 and 15 years and commonly affects young adults. Their symptoms may be confused with DMD as the children often have an exaggerated lumbar lordosis, hip abductor and extensor weakness, and a positive Trendelenburg sign. Knee extensor weakness and hyperextension are also

seen. Walking deteriorates in late adolescence and most are wheelchair users in adult life although life expectancy is usually normal.

Further Investigations

Muscle biopsies reveal a typical neuropathic pattern and EMG shows characteristic fibrillation and fasciculation potentials.

The genetic locus for SMA has been identified on chromosome 5q [8]. In 96% of patients autosomal recessive SMA is caused by mutation of the survival motor neurone gene (SMN1). SMN1 can also be replaced by an almost identical gene, SMN2, also located on the same chromosome. Deletions within both copies of SMN1 result in Type 1 SMA (Werdnig–Hoffmann) and the milder forms of SMA result when SMN1 is replaced by SMN2 [9–12]. Boylan et al. [13] have described a rare form of SMA that is inherited in an autosomal dominant pattern.

Orthopaedic Management

Scoliosis in SMA develops early and invariably progresses to a severe degree. Posterior spinal fusion and instrumentation should be performed relatively early in the non-walker before the curve becomes too severe. Early post-operative management can be challenging because of respiratory compromise so anterior spinal surgery should be avoided. Spinal fusion in walkers may remove compensatory lumbar and pelvic movement and reduce their walking ability.

Contractures of the hip and knee are inevitable in the non-walker and there is no functional gain from surgical releases at the hip or knee as any improvement is difficult to maintain and recurrence of the deformities is the norm. Hip displacement is common in SMA and coxa valga is often seen radiologically. Attempts to relocate hips have not been very satisfactory and Zenios et al. [14] concluded that surgery for subluxation of the hip in SMA is not justified. Sporer and Smith [15] noted that a small number of patients had symptoms associated with dislocated hips and recommended observation rather than surgery in these patients.

Muscular Dystrophies

The general distribution of muscle weakness in the commoner dystrophies is shown in Fig. 3.9 [16].

Duchenne Type

The prevalence of this sex-linked, severe, and progressive dystrophy has been estimated at between 1.9 and 3.4 per 100,000 of the population. It is a disease almost entirely exclusive to males. Female carriers can be detected by an increased serum CK concentration in 70–75% of cases. Delay in motor milestones or clumsiness in a boy are the usual presentations of DMD.

Further Investigations

Dystrophin, the protein missing in DMD, is also expressed in the brain and occasionally the boys may first present with a delay in intellectual development, as their mean IQ is less than their peers [17]. Any boy not walking by 18 months, with global developmental delay, or with delayed speech development should have their serum CK level checked. The diagnosis is confirmed by genetic testing for the deletion in the Xp21 gene that encodes for dystrophin, which is absent in DMD, thus avoiding the need for muscle biopsy. Spontaneous mutations occur in approximately 30% of new cases of DMD.

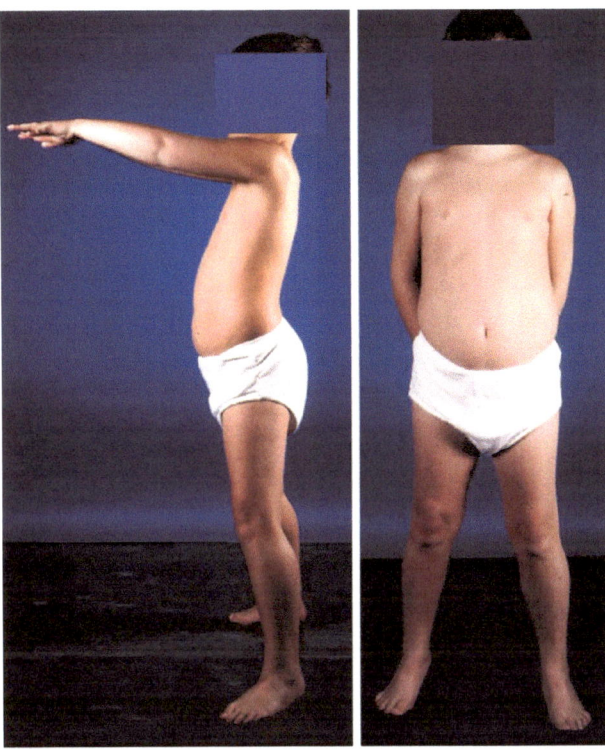

Fig. 3.10 Duchenne muscular dystrophy. Note the prominent abdomen and lumbar lordosis, calf pseudohypertrophy, and equinus at the ankles

Clinical Features

The earliest symptoms are clumsiness, impaired balance, and a tiptoe gait because of the muscle weakness (Fig. 3.10). Muscle hypotonia and pseudohypertrophy is usually seen and sometimes the boy first presents as a toe walker because of muscle weakness. Although present at birth, the disease does not normally manifest itself until the age of 3–4 years. Walking ceases at a median age of 10 years (range 7–11 years); fatal respiratory failure occurs between the ages of 19 and 21 years and occasionally up to 25 years. The intellect is affected, and approximately 30% of patients have an intelligence quotient (IQ) less than 75.

Orthopaedic Management

Obesity is common in the muscular dystrophies, probably as a result of immobility. The condition is incurable; attempts have been made to slow its rate of progress with steroid therapy, which has benefited some boys if used before the onset of weakness. However, the side effects of steroids such as weight gain, cataracts, and osteoporosis may outweigh the benefits. Although cardiac muscle is involved, symptomatic cardiomyopathy is unusual, unlike in BMD and Friedrich's ataxia. Survival is improving and advances in gene therapy may offer improved prospects for patients in the future.

Most boys with DMD develop scoliosis, typically a long C-shaped curve and associated pelvic obliquity. This is often associated with hyperlordosis due to hip flexion contractures. The pelvic obliquity may be associated with hip displacement [18]. The scoliosis deteriorates after cessation of walking and often causes difficulties in comfortable seating and skin pressure care where there is rib impingement against the iliac crest. It is generally considered that scoliosis should be treated surgically in DMD [19] although, to date, there are no randomized controlled clinical trials available to evaluate its effectiveness and thus no evidence-based recommendation can be made for clinical practice [20]. However, the clinical impression is that patients benefit from spinal surgery performed early, before the combination of a progressing deformity and deteriorating respiratory function becomes an unacceptable surgical risk. Surgery should be considered once the Cobb angle has reached 30° and before the forced vital capacity is less than 35% of age-matched normal values [21]. Pre-operative cardiac and pulmonary assessments are mandatory and the surgery should be carried out in a center where there is appropriate expertise. The surgery comprises posterior spinal fusion with instrumentation and segmental stabilization using either pedicle screw fixation or segmental sublaminar wiring, or a combination of both. Anterior surgical approaches that divide the diaphragm should be avoided because of impaired respiratory function. Fixation to the pelvis is recommended to provide a level pelvis for comfortable seating. Complications of spinal surgery in DMD are a concern; blood loss is generally higher than that for equivalent surgery in idiopathic scoliosis and Shapiro and Sethna [22] and Ramirez et al. [23]. have reported complication rates of 27%. Velasco et al. [24] showed that the rates of respiratory decline were 4% per year pre-surgery and decreased to 1.75% per year after posterior spinal fusion.

The extensive release of contractures to prolong walking beyond the usual age of 10 years (when it ceases in most boys who have DMD) must be very selective. Claims that boys of 14 or 15 years continue to walk after surgical treatment have to be questioned, because they may have had undiagnosed BMD. In addition, there is a variation in the age at which the ability to walk in DMD is lost so this is a confounding factor when considering the effect of surgery in prolonging the ability to walk. After surgery the period of walking is generally brief, as energy consumption is too great. Helping the patient achieve optimal function and independence in a powered wheelchair and with adaptations to other equipments is probably more appropriate in the longer term.

There is no indication to release hip and knee contractures in non-walkers with DMD. However, equino-varus deformities of the feet can be treated surgically when there is difficulty in the shoe fitting or pressure symptoms over the lateral border of the foot when it rests on the footplate of the wheelchair. This can be managed by lengthening of the tendo-Achilles and tibialis posterior. The equinus is not necessarily confined to the ankle and if a fixed plantaris deformity is present it requires bony surgery for correction. Usually this component of the equinus can be accepted and managed with an orthosis to avoid extensive surgery in a boy with respiratory compromise.

Although DMD affects the upper limbs they do not require surgical intervention.

Prognosis

Death from progressive respiratory failure usually occurs by the late teens to early twenties and once the vital capacity falls below 1 l the 5-year survival rate is only 8% [25]. Home ventilation has improved survival and Dreher et al. [26]. reported a median survival of 132 months after beginning mechanical home ventilation in 12 patients with DMD. Recent improvements in survival are probably due to better management of chest infections, correction of the scoliosis, and non-invasive ventilation. With advances in gene therapy it is possible that the life expectancy for boys with DMD will be further improved.

Benign X-Linked (Becker) Muscular Dystrophy

Clinical Signs

BMD is a sex-linked recessive muscle disease that differs from DMD by its later onset and relatively benign course. Only 10% of those affected cease to walk before the age of 40 years. Calf enlargement is the most frequent early sign of the disease and muscle cramps are more common than in the other dystrophies and myopathies. Leg pains and cramps are so prevalent in childhood that patients with BMD can be mistaken for having non-specific leg pains or cramp after exercise.

Diagnosis

Serum CK is high and a normal finding rules it out in boys who complain of persistent leg pains and cramps. Muscle dystrophin determination will differentiate BMD from DMD because dystrophin is present, albeit in smaller amounts than normal, in the former and absent in the latter. About 85% of males with BMD have an identifiable mutation in the DMD gene. Bushy, Thambyayah, and Gardner-Medwin [27] have shown that the prevalence rate of BMD is 2.38 per 100,000 compared to 2.48 per 100,000 for DMD. The cumulative birth incidence of BMD (at least 1 in 18,450 male live births) is about one-third that of DMD (1 in 5,618 male live births), suggesting that BMD is more common than previously thought.

Prognosis

Contractures are rare and do not occur until very late in the disease when the patient is already confined to a wheelchair. Life expectancy exceeds that of DMD (mean age of death 42 years, range 23–63 years) but patients are at risk of cardiomyopathy.

Emery–Dreifuss Muscular Dystrophy

Emery–Dreifuss muscular dystrophy (EDMD) was first described in 1966 [28] and its inheritance is usually X-linked but can also be autosomal dominant. The gene associated with EDMD is located in the distal Xq28 region of the X chromosome [29] and encodes for a nuclear membrane protein, emerin [30, 31]. Recent studies have shown that alterations in lamins, the principal component of the nuclear lamina, have been found in a phenotype resembling EDMD

[32], which may account for the cardiac conduction system disease seen in EDMD.

Clinical Signs

EDMD is characterized by a triad of features: (1) early contractures of the Achilles tendons, elbows, and post-cervical muscles; (2) slowly progressive muscle wasting and weakness with a predominantly humero-peroneal distribution in the early stages; and (3) cardiomyopathy with conduction defects and risk of sudden death [28, 29]. The initial presentation of EDMD is a non-specific muscle weakness in the first few years of life, with an awkward gait and, possibly, toe-walking. The dystrophy becomes fully developed in the second decade of life and, most importantly, these patients have bradycardia and eventually develop complete heart block which may be silent.

The serum CK concentration is only slightly to moderately elevated and levels are not as high as those seen in DMD or BMD. If the latter have been ruled out by dystrophin estimation the diagnosis of EDMD should be considered.

Prognosis

Muscle weakness is progressive but slow, so that walking is generally possible until the fifth or sixth decades of life. The ankle equinus can become severe. Elbow contractures appear as early as 7 years, whereas limited flexion of the neck caused by the extension contracture may be evident at 5 years and is clearly present by the twenties. The importance of defining this type of muscular dystrophy is the need for a cardiac assessment. Bradycardia and a first-degree atrio-ventricular heart block can result in sudden death between the ages of 25 and 60 years [33].

Orthopaedic Management

Lengthening of the Achilles tendon may be indicated for severe equinus. If varus of the foot is present, lengthening or transfer of the posterior tibial tendon may be indicated. Elbow flexion contracture, even if it is 90°, rarely limits function; consequently, no treatment is necessary as further flexion, pronation, and supination are usually preserved. If scoliosis develops, it generally stabilizes at an acceptable 40° after spinal growth has ceased, so that surgery is probably not indicated. The cervical extension contracture limits neck flexion and later there may be a restriction of lateral rotation as well.

Limb-Girdle Muscular Dystrophies

Limb-girdle muscular dystrophy (LGMD) is a descriptive term for a spectrum of inherited muscle disorders that have a fairly similar phenotype [34]. They are characterized by progressive muscle wasting and weakness of variable distribution and severity [16, 35]. These are distinct from DMD and BMD and the commoner types have an autosomal recessive inheritance but the spectrum also includes rare subtypes that have an autosomal dominant inheritance pattern. The molecular genetics of this spectrum of disorders is complex and numerous abnormalities have been identified but are beyond the scope of this chapter.

Clinical Signs

Two broad patterns are seen; those that affect the upper limbs in adolescence (scapulo-humeral type) and those that affect the lower limbs (limb-girdle type), without facial weakness, after the age of 20 years. In more severe cases, the distal muscles of the limbs are also affected. The presence of facial weakness changes the term to fascio-scapulo-humeral (FSH) muscular dystrophy. The hallmark of the scapulo-humeral type of LGMD is winging of the scapula (Fig. 3.11). Although the biceps and triceps are affected the deltoid seems to be preserved. Foot drop as a result of anterior tibial muscle weakness occurs in the FSH type, but is rare in the scapulo-humeral form. Contractures of muscles and joints are not a prominent feature.

An infantile form of FSH muscular dystrophy has been identified. It is more severe than the adult form and is inherited as an autosomal recessive. Facial diplegia and sensorineural hearing loss are usually diagnosed by the age of 5 years. Scapular winging is present but the most striking deformity is a marked lumbar lordosis, upon which

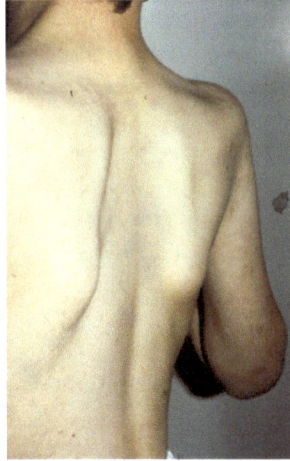

Fig. 3.11 Winging of the scapula in scapulo-humeral dystrophy. Courtesy of Dr P. Eunson

the patient depends to maintain balance. Walking ability is usually lost after the age of 20 years [33].

Diagnosis

The CK concentration is very high in the LGMDs and EMG confirms a general myopathy. A normal dystrophin assay will distinguish LGMD from DMD and BMD.

Orthopaedic Management

General measures include weight control, exercise to maintain mobility, and the prevention of contractures. Specifically, scapulothoracic fusion may be indicated for intractable pain, loss of range of shoulder movement, and scapular instability during upper limb tasks. Berne et al. [36] found that abduction increased by 25° and flexion increased 29° at a nearly 10-year average follow-up after scapulothoracic fusion in patients with FSH muscular dystrophy. However, Krishnan et al. [37] have reported complications in more than half of their 22 patients after scapulothoracic fusion.

Scoliosis rarely requires spinal fusion because the onset of the disease is later than that of DMD. Severe lordosis is more common than scoliosis and there may be no useful solution other than recommending a wheelchair if it causes intractable back pain. Attempts to correct the lordosis by spinal fusion will remove the ability to balance so that standing and walking will become impossible.

A leaf spring AFO may be useful in controlling a foot drop provided there is no fixed deformity at the ankle and it remains mobile.

Congenital Muscular Dystrophy

The congenital muscular dystrophies (CMDs) are a group of disorders almost all of which are inherited in an autosomal recessive manner. There are syndromic and non-syndromic types of CMD and in the former structural abnormalities of the brain are seen on an MRI scan. The infants are floppy at birth and may also have joint contractures. The serum CK is usually elevated and muscle biopsy shows a dystrophic or myopathic pattern. In contrast to DMD and BMD, no involvement of the dystrophin gene is found.

Merosin deficiency of the basement membrane has been shown to cause CMD linked to chromosome 6q2 and merosin CMD is prevalent in European populations. In Japan mutation of the fukutin gene has been identified in the majority of cases of Fukuyama CMD [38].

Muscle Myopathies

The myopathies are characterized by hypotonia at birth (the floppy infant) and by delay in motor development. In childhood and adolescence, joint contractures, foot deformities, and scoliosis are common as the disease progresses. The varieties of myopathy can be diagnosed only by muscle biopsy and histological studies. Serum enzymes are within normal limits, and EMG shows only the non-specific electrical activity of myopathies in general.

Central Core Disease

This has a wide spectrum of clinical presentation and is usually inherited as an autosomal dominant condition although autosomal recessive cases are also seen. In milder cases most children achieve independent walking and their life expectancy is usually normal. In severe cases children present with profound hypotonia, scoliosis, and hip dislocation, succumbing to respiratory failure early in life. This disorder may cause unexpected outcomes in children who are being treated for presumed developmental dysplasia of the hip as redislocation occurs in more than 50% of cases. Recurrent dislocation of the patella is resistant to surgical correction and pes planus is very common. Scoliosis can be managed with instrumentation and fusion.

The diagnosis is made on muscle biopsy where typical cores are seen and most cases are associated with a mutation in RYR1 that codes for ryanodine receptor 1. Surgeons and anesthetists should be aware that patients who have central core myopathy are prone to malignant hyperthermia [39].

Nemaline Myopathy

This is a rare disorder that can be inherited either in an autosomal dominant or recessive manner (Fig. 3.12). There is a wide spectrum of clinical presentation. Hypotonia is associated with unusually slender, but reportedly surprisingly strong, muscles. The distribution of weakness is seen mainly in the face, flexors of the neck, and proximal limbs. Facial weakness and nasal speech are the results of palatal muscle weakness. Scoliosis, hypermobility, and foot deformities are common but disability from muscle weakness is only moderate. Feeding difficulties and respiratory failure as a result of diaphragmatic involvement are seen. The diagnosis is made on muscle biopsy where nemaline rods are seen in the sarcoplasm of skeletal muscle fibers. No definitive correlation

Fig. 3.12 Nemaline myopathy.
Courtesy of Dr P. Eunson

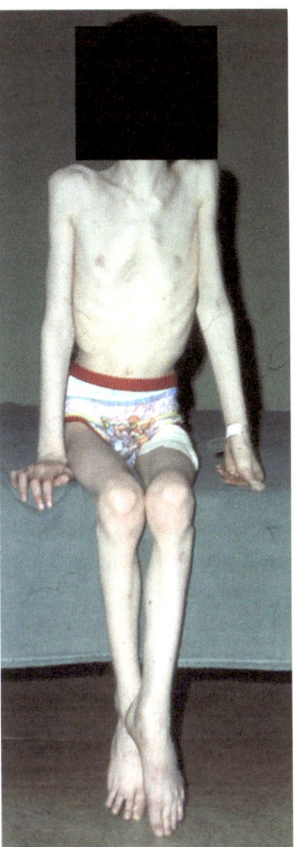

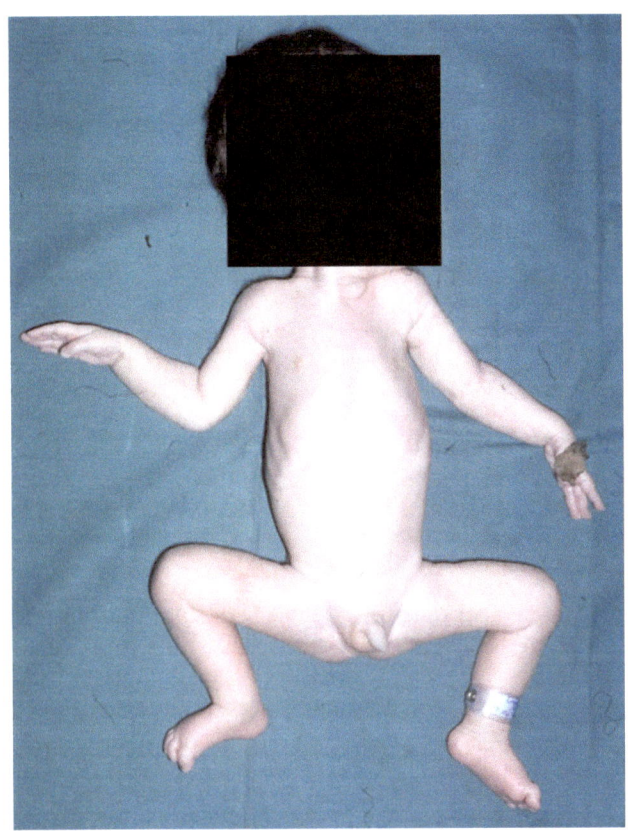

Fig. 3.13   Myotubular myopathy. Courtesy of Dr P. Eunson

has been found between the number of rods and severity or age of onset of the myopathy [40].

X-linked Myotubular Myopathy, Congenital Fiber-Type Disproportion, Multiminicore Disease, and Mitochondrial Disease

Congenital fiber-type disproportion is a genetically heterogeneous condition and mitochondrial diseases are a clinically heterogeneous group of disorders that arise as a result of dysfunction of the mitochondrial respiratory chain [41]. Multiminicore disease is inherited in an autosomal recessive manner and X-linked myotubular myopathy (Fig. 3.13) is associated with a mutation in MTM1. These myopathies have no distinctive clinical features other than hypotonia, muscle weakness, contractures, and scoliosis.

Myotonias

Clinical Signs

Myotonia is muscle contraction that persists after the voluntary effort has ended. The muscle relaxes slowly, so that a handshake, for example, gives the sensation of a lingering grip.

Diagnosis

Diagnosis is confirmed by the EMG pattern, which depicts the initial contraction of the muscle with a gradual trailing-off in activity (Fig. 3.14).

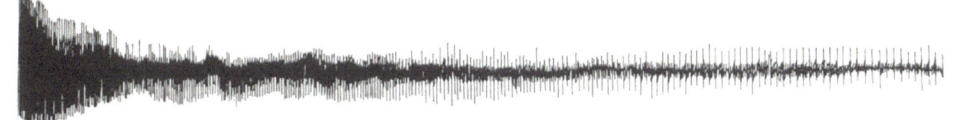

Fig. 3.14 Electromyograph showing classic myotonic discharge pattern on voluntary muscle contraction

Fig. 3.15 Myotonia congenita.
Courtesy of Dr P. Eunson

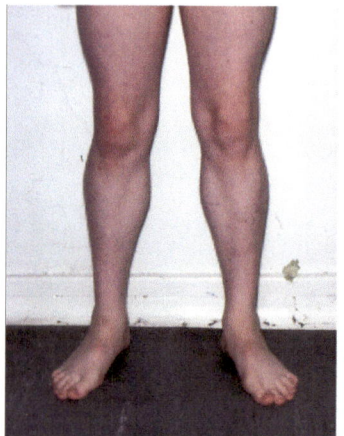
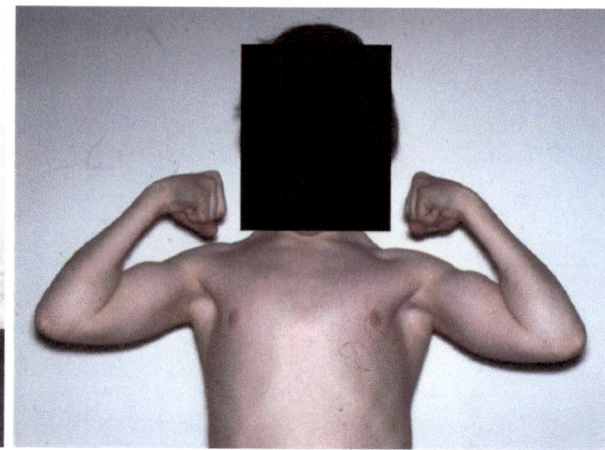

Myotonia Congenita

Myotonia congenita usually affects infants. The symptoms of stiffness are made worse by rest and cold but are relieved by exercise. The patients are strong and have well-developed muscles (Fig. 3.15). Surgeons and anesthetists should be aware that these children are prone to malignant hyperthermia and depolarizing muscle relaxants should be avoided. Myotonia congenita is inherited both in an autosomal recessive manner (Becker disease) and in an autosomal dominant manner (Thomsen disease). The diagnosis is made on clinical examination, EMG (which shows myotonic bursts of activity), and a family history. A mutation of CLCN1 is associated with myotonia congenita [42].

Myotonic Dystrophy

Two forms are recognized: type 1, also known as Steinert disease, and type 2 or proximal myotonic myopathy. Both have autosomal dominant inheritance patterns. Rare, as muscle diseases are, type 1 has an incidence of 4.9–5.5 per 100,000 of the population. The genetic defect in type 1 is a mutation in chromosome 19 and in type 2 in chromosome 3 in some patients. There is a spectrum of phenotypes in type 1 from mild to severe and type 2 generally affects adults.

Congenital Myotonic Dystrophy

Infants with congenital myotonic dystrophy have severe hypotonia at birth, facial diplegia, a long narrow face, mental retardation, and a high incidence of severe clubfoot. Characteristically, they experience difficulty in breathing and feeding. All affected children present with delays in speech and motor development, but eventually walk. The clinical signs are fully developed by the time the child is aged 10 years, and some develop scoliosis in adolescence.

Polymyositis–Dermatomyositis

Polymyositis and dermatomyositis do occur in children and represent a spectrum of autoimmune disease [43]. Dermatomyositis is the most frequent inflammatory myopathy in children but polymyositis is rare. In dermatomyositis, a butterfly-shaped rash on the anterior neck and upper chest, hyperemia at the base of the fingernails, and shiny red skin at the pulps of the fingers are important clues to diagnosis. In late cases, radiographs of the limb may show tiny flecks and plaques of calcification in the muscles and under the skin. Polymyositis should be considered in children presenting with unexplained gradual muscle weakness and difficulty in elevating the arms or climbing stairs. It is important to exclude a muscle dystrophy and the diagnosis of polymyositis is one of the exclusion. Serum CK is markedly raised in polymyositis and may be elevated in dermatomyositis. EMG shows myopathic changes and MRI may show increased signal in affected muscles but is non-specific. Muscle biopsy will show degeneration, regeneration, and infiltration with inflammatory cells. The child should be referred to a paediatric rheumatologist.

Myasthenia Gravis

The characteristic presenting feature of myasthenia gravis is painless, fatigable weakness either developing or becoming more evident with exertion [44]. The condition is very rare in children and forms a heterogeneous group of diseases that are caused by an abnormality of neuromuscular transmission. This may be considered as pre-synaptic (e.g., an abnormality of choline acetyltransferase), synaptic, or post-synaptic (e.g., an abnormality of the acetylcholine receptor) [45]. In congenital myasthenia the infant may present with a bulbar palsy and respiratory distress.

In later life symptoms are generally insidious in onset and often variable. The patient may initially experience ptosis and diplopia from involvement of the facial muscles and then pharyngeal muscle weakness causes difficulties with speech and swallowing. The symptoms may progress to include general muscular weakness or the patient may present with respiratory arrest. The importance to surgeons and anesthetists is that myasthenic patients are sensitive to non-depolarizing muscle relaxants.

Acknowledgments We thank Dr Paul Eunson, consultant paediatric neurologist, Royal Hospital for Sick Children Edinburgh, for his helpful suggestions in the preparation of this chapter and for providing many of the clinical illustrations, and Dr Colin Smith, senior lecturer in pathology, University of Edinburgh, for providing the histological illustrations.

References

1. Read L, Galasko CSB. Delay in diagnosing Duchenne muscular dystrophy in orthopaedic clinics. J Bone Joint Surg Br 1986; 68:481–482.
2. Gowda V, Parr J, Jayawant S. Evaluation of the floppy infant. Paediatr Child Health 2008; 18:17–21.
3. André T, Chesni Y, St Anne-Dargassies A. The neurological examination of the infant. Little Club Clinics in Developmental Medicine No 1. Spastics Society 1960.
4. Dubowitz V. The Floppy Infant, 2nd ed. Clinics In Developmental Medicine. Mac Keith Press, London; 1980.
5. Gardner-Medwin D, Hudgson P, Walton JN. Benign spinal muscular atrophy arising in childhood and adolescence. J Neurol Sci 1967; 5:121–158.
6. Evans GA, Drennan J, Russman BS. Functional classification and orthopaedic management of spinal muscular atrophy. J Bone Joint Surg Br 1981; 63B:516–522.
7. Gamble JG, Rinsky LA, Lee JH. Orthopaedic aspects of central core disease. J Bone Joint Surg Am 1988; 70: 1061–1066.
8. Brzustowicz LM, Lehner T, Castilla LH, et al. Genetic mapping of chronic childhood-onset spinal muscular atrophy to chromosome 5q11.2–13.3. Nature 1990; 344:540–541.
9. Lefebvre S, Burglen L, Reboullet S, et al. Identification and characterization of a spinal muscular atrophy-determining gene. Cell 1995; 80:155–165.
10. Swoboda KJ, Prior TW, Scott CB, et al. Natural history of denervation in SMA: relation to age, SMN2 copy number, and function. Ann Neurol 2005; 57:704–712.
11. Yamashita M, Nishio H, Harada Y, et al. Significant increase in the number of the SMN2 gene copies in an adult-onset type III spinal muscular atrophy patient with homozygous deletion of the NAIP gene. Eur Neurol 2004; 52:101–106.
12. Sumner CJ. Molecular mechanisms of spinal muscular atrophy. J Child Neurol 2007; 22:979–989.
13. Boylan KB, Cornblath DR, Glass JD, et al. Autosomal dominant distal spinal muscular atrophy in four generations. Neurology 1995; 45:699–704.
14. Zenios M, Sampath J, Cole C, et al. Operative treatment for hip subluxation in spinal muscular atrophy. J Bone Joint Surg Br 2005; 87B:1541–1544.
15. Sporer SM, Smith BG. Hip dislocation in patients with spinal muscular atrophy. J Pediatr Orthop 2003; 23:10–14.
16. Emery AE. The muscle dystrophies. Lancet 2002; 359(9307): 687–695.
17. Zwelleger H, Hanson JW. Psychometric studies in muscular dystrophy type IIIa (Duchenne). Dev Med Child Neurol 1967; 9:576–581.
18. Chan KG, Galasko CSB, Delaney C. Hip subluxation and dislocation in Duchenne muscular dystrophy. J Pediatr Orthop Br 2001; 10:219–225.
19. Kinali M, Messina S, Mercuri E, et al. Management of scoliosis in Duchenne muscular dystrophy: a large 10-year retrospective study. Dev Med Child Neurol 2006; 48:513–518.
20. Cheuk DK, Wong V, Wraige E, et al. Surgery for scoliosis in Duchenne muscular dystrophy. Cochrane Database Syst Rev 2007; Jan 24(1):CD005375.
21. Miller RG, Chalmers AC, Dao H, et al. The effect of spine fusion on respiratory function in Duchenne muscular dystrophy. Neurology 1991; 41:38–40.
22. Shapiro F, Sethna N. Blood loss in pediatric spine surgery. Eur Spine J 2004; 13 Suppl 1:S6–S17.
23. Ramirez N, Richards BS, Warren PD, Williams GR. Complications after posterior spinal fusion in Duchenne's muscular dystrophy. J Pediatr Orthop 1997; 17:109–114.
24. Velasco MV, Colin AA, Zurakowski D, et al. Posterior spinal fusion for scoliosis in Duchenne muscular dystrophy diminishes the rate of respiratory decline. Spine 2007; 32:459–465.
25. Phillips MF, Quinlivan RC, Edwards RH, Calverley PM. Changes in spirometry over time as a prognostic marker in patients with Duchenne muscular dystrophy. Am J Respir Crit Care Med 2001; 164:2191–2194.
26. Dreher M, Rauter I, Storre JH, et al. When should home mechanical ventilation be started in patients with different neuromuscular disorders? Respirology 2007; 12:749–753.
27. Bushby KM, Thambyayah M, Gardner-Medwin D. Prevalence and incidence of Becker muscular dystrophy. Lancet 1991; 337:1022–1024.
28. Emery AE, Dreifuss FE. Unusual type of benign x-linked muscular dystrophy. J Neurol Neurosurg Psychiatr 1966; 29:338–342.
29. Yates JR, Warner JP, Smith JA, et al. Emery-Dreifuss muscular dystrophy: linkage to markers in distal Xq28. J Med Genet 1993; 30:108–111.
30. Manilal S, Nguyen TM, Sewry CA, Morris GE. The Emery-Dreifuss muscular dystrophy protein. Hum Mol Genet 1996; 5:801–808.
31. Ura S, Hayashi YK, Goto K, et al. Limb-girdle muscular dystrophy due to emerin gene mutations. Arch Neurol 2007; 64:1038–1041.
32. Maioli MA, Marrosu G, Mateddu A, et al. A novel mutation in the central rod domain of lamin A/C producing a phenotype resembling the Emery-Dreifuss muscular dystrophy phenotype. Muscle Nerve 2007; 36:828–832.
33. Shapiro F, Specht L. Current Concepts Review. The diagnosis and orthopaedic treatment of inherited muscular diseases of childhood. J Bone Joint Surg Am 1993; 75A:439–454.
34. Mathews KD, Moore SA. Limb-girdle muscular dystrophy. Curr Neurol Neurosci Rep 2003; 3:78–85.
35. Emery AEH. Fortnightly review: The muscular dystrophies. Br Med J 1998; 317:991–995.
36. Berne D, Laude F, Laporte C, et al. Scapulothoracic arthrodesis in facioscapulohumeral muscular dystrophy. Clin Orth Rel Res 2003; 409:106–113.

37. Krishnan SG, Hawkins RJ, Michelotti JD, et al. Scapulothoracic arthrodesis: indications, technique, and results. Clin Orthop Rel Res 2005; 435:126–133.

38. Tomé FM. The Peter Emil Becker Award lecture 1998. The saga of congenital muscular dystrophy. Neuropediatrics 1999; 30:55–65.

39. Treves S, Jungbluth H, Muntoni F, Zorzato F. Congenital muscle disorders with cores: the ryanodine receptor calcium channel paradigm. Curr Opin Pharmacol 2008; 8(3):319–326.

40. Ryan MM, Ilkovski B, Strickland CD, et al. Clinical course correlates poorly with muscle pathology in nemaline myopathy. Neurology 2003; 60:665–673.

41. Wallace DC. Mitochondrial diseases in man and mouse. Science 1999; 283:1482–1488.

42. Colding-Jørgensen E. Phenotypic variability in myotonia congenital. Muscle Nerve 2005; 32:19–34.

43. Ramanan AV, Feldman BM. Clinical features of juvenile dermatomyositis and other childhood onset myositis syndromes. Rheum Dis Clin N Am 2002; 28:833–857.

44. Vincent A, Palace J, Hilton-Jones D. Myasthenia gravis. Lancet 2001; 357:2122–2128.

45. Hantai D, Richard P, Koenig J, Eymard B. Congenital myasthenic syndromes. Curr Opin Neurol 2004; 17:539–551.

Chapter 4

Neural Tube Defects, Spina Bifida, and Spinal Dysraphism

H. Kerr Graham and Klaus Parsch

Introduction

Neural tube defects are a varied group of congenital spinal anomalies associated with abnormal closure of the neural tube. Anencephaly represents the most severe abnormality that may occur at the cranial end of the tube.

Spina bifida is the general term used to describe conditions caused by disturbance of the development of the vertebral arches. They are often associated with abnormalities of the structures derived from the neural tube and the meninges and may be associated with cyst formation.

Spinal dysraphism refers to a number of hidden abnormalities affecting the spinal cord or cauda equina which may produce occult or overt neurological disturbance. The diversity of these conditions suggests that causative factors exert their effects at different periods of fetal development.

The absence of the posterior elements of spine allows for the extrusion of the meninges (meningocele) and the spinal cord elements (myelomeningocele). Lesions in the cervical spine tend to be meningoceles and are often associated with other defects like the Arnold–Chiari malformation.

Myelomeningocele

The exposed cord and neurons seem to function early in gestation but are progressively destroyed (Fig. 4.1). This has prompted the development of intrauterine surgery to close the defect in an attempt to limit neurological deterioration. Some early results are encouraging. Myelomeningocele remains the form of neural tube defect which most commonly leads to spinal deformity with significant motor and sensory deficit in the lower limbs.

H.K. Graham (✉)
Department of Orthopaedics, The Royal Children's Hospital, Parkville, Victoria, Australia

In addition to the major spinal defect, other lesions are frequently present—the Arnold–Chiari malformation (cerebellum and brainstem displaced distally and compressed at the foramen magnum), cerebellar hypoplasia, hydrocephalus, hydromyelia, syringomyelia, and diastematomyelia. Many patients also have upper limb problems due to a variety of subtle neurological lesions which may prove progressive. Children with myelomeningocele generally have paralysis of the bladder, bowel incontinence, and a propensity to trophic ulceration in areas of insensate skin. Approximately 80% of affected children will develop hydrocephalus and as a group these children score 10–15 points below average on standardized intelligence tests. Neuropsychological testing reveals a consistent profile of learning difficulties and short-term memory problems, as well as deficits in visuospatial, perceptual, numerical, and executive skills.

Spina Bifida

Incidence

The incidence of spina bifida varies with the geographical area and ethnicity. There are also seasonal variations. During the past 20 years there has been a dramatic decrease in the number of births of children with spina bifida in developed countries and a less dramatic fall in the incidence of pregnancies with spina bifida. Peri-conceptual vitamin supplementation, maternal alpha-fetoprotein testing, routine antenatal ultrasound, and termination of affected pregnancies are some of the factors which have brought about this change.

The highest incidence in the world was reported in Ireland, Wales, and the north of England (up to 5 per 1000 live births), although this has now dropped precipitously. A high incidence has been reported in certain regions of China. In North America and Australia the incidence is less than 1 per 1000 live births.

Fig. 4.1 (**a**) A newborn child with an open spina bifida lesion and dressing in situ. Evidence of congenital deformities and muscle imbalance can be seen and much gained by careful neonatal examination. (**b**) The sites of neurological involvement include hydrocephalus, the Chiari 2 malformation, syringomyelia, and the tethered cord. While the problems of hydrocephalus are generally seen neonatally, neurological deterioration secondary to the Chiari 2 malformation, syringomyelia, and cord tethering often present insidiously in later childhood

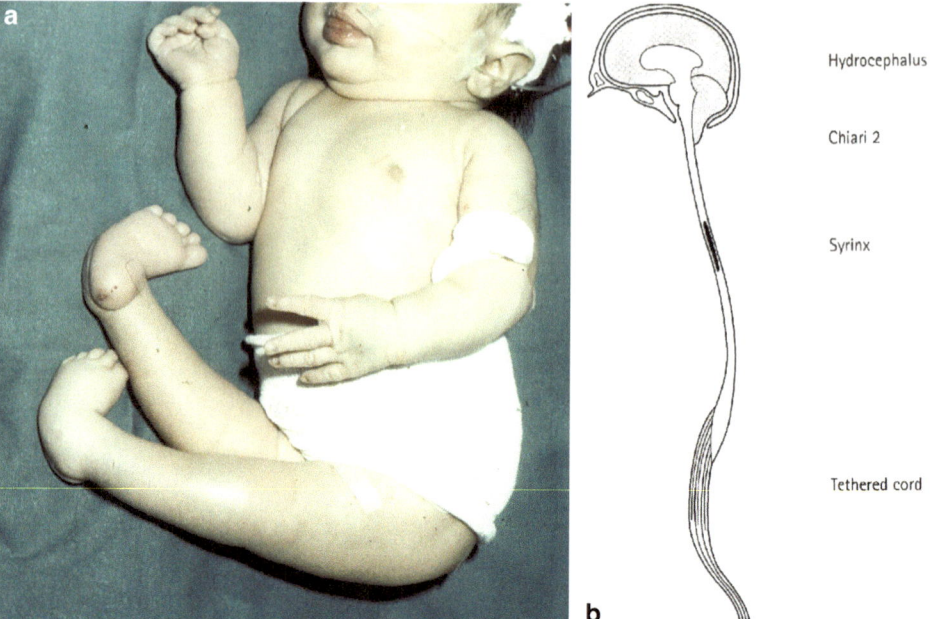

Etiology

This is thought to be multifactorial and both genetic and environmental factors have been implicated. It is believed that the spectrum of neural tube defects results from similar causes acting at slightly different times during embryogenesis.

Genetic Predisposition

Neural tube defects have been shown to follow a multifactorial pattern of inheritance. A number of genes are thought to have a small additive effect which may combine with environmental factors. When this compound effect passes a critical threshold the child is liable to be born with a neural tube defect. There is also an association with chromosomal disorders (trisomy 13, trisomy 18, triploidy, unbalanced translocations, and microdeletion of 22q11) as well as rare dominant and recessive disorders. Recently, substances that interfere with the GABA receptors have been implicated. The birth of a child with spina bifida predisposes to subsequent children being born with anencephaly, with extensive congenital vertebral abnormalities or with spinal dysraphism.

Diet and Drugs

The environmental factors which have been suggested as a cause of neural tube defects include folate deficiency, other vitamin deficiencies, absence of selenium from the regional soil and hence from the diet, poor maternal nutrition, a high maternal alcohol intake, maternal diabetes mellitus, fever at a

critical stage of pregnancy, and a wide variety of other factors [1]. Drugs associated with an increased incidence of neural tube defects include anti-epileptic agents such as sodium valproate and carbamazepine, isotretinoin (for the treatment of acne), etretinate (for the treatment of psoriasis), thalidomide, and methotrexate.

Embryology and Pathology

Spina bifida may be subdivided into spina bifida cystica, when a cyst forms, and spina bifida occulta, when the defect is completely or largely hidden from the examining eye. The various forms of spina bifida are illustrated in Fig. 4.2.

Spina Bifida Cystica

This can occur in the following forms:

Myeloschisis or myelocele (Fig. 4.2a). The vertebral arches are deficient and neural plate material is spread out on the surface, sometimes in a shallow depression, more commonly over a cystic swelling of the meninges.

Myelomeningocele (Fig. 4.2b). There is a fluid-filled cystic swelling, lined by dura and arachnoid, protruding through a defect in the vertebral arches under the skin. The spinal cord and nerve roots are carried out into the fundus of the sac.

Meningocele (Fig. 4.2c). There is a cystic swelling of dura and arachnoid, protruding through a defect in the vertebral arches under the skin. The spinal cord is entirely confined within the vertebral arches but may exhibit abnormalities.

Fig. 4.2 Schematic diagrams of the major types of spina bifida. (**a**) Myeloschisis; (**b**) myelomeningocele; (**c**) meningocele; and (**d**) spina bifida occulta

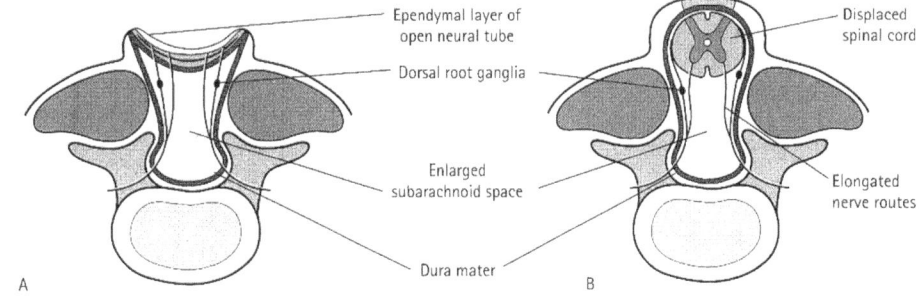

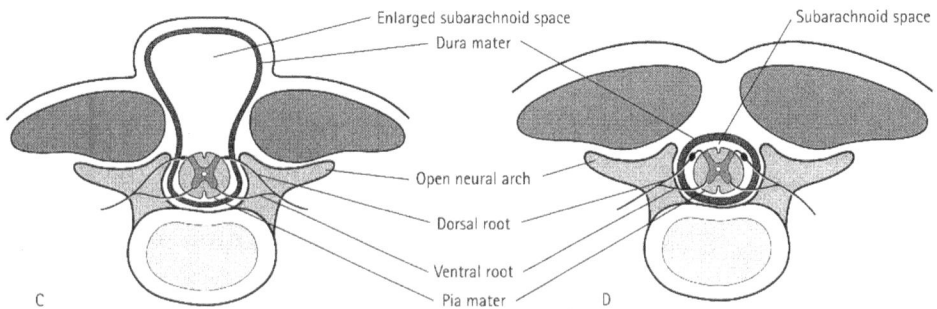

Spina Bifida Occulta

In this form (Fig. 4.2d), there is a localized defect in one or more of the vertebral arches, because the respective halves of the vertebral arches fail to meet and fuse in the third month of intrauterine life. The spinal cord and meninges remain within the vertebral canal. The skin overlying the spina bifida occulta may be normal or there may be a dimple which may be connected with the dura by a fibrous cord, a patch of hair, pigmentation, or a lipoma (possibly continuous with a similar intradural lipoma). All these and the rare intramedullary dermoid probably represent abnormalities of separation of presumptive skin from neural tissue, as both are ectodermal in origin, during the process of closure of the neural tube. These conditions will be considered under the heading "spinal dysraphism."

Causes of Deformity

Muscle Imbalance Due to Lower Motor Neurone Lesions

Muscle imbalance has been traditionally regarded as the major cause of deformity in patients with spina bifida. However, it is only one of many causes and may be less important than suggested by some earlier studies. The imbalance is due in large part to the defects in the nerve roots and spinal cord already present at birth. However, further neurological injury, associated with a change in neurosegmental

level, may be produced by prenatal traction on the abnormally tethered cord, direct pressure and longitudinal shearing forces during delivery, and postnatal drying and infection of the neural plate [1]. There is some correlation between the lowest functioning neurosegmental level, the muscles acting, and the limb posture (Table 4.1). This correlation is most obvious at the foot and ankle but less so at the hip. Patients in whom L5 is spared almost invariably have a calcaneus deformity of the foot because of activity in the tibialis anterior, the peroneus tertius, and the extensor digitorum longus, and no activity in the soleus or gastrocnemius. Such muscle imbalance ultimately leads to fixed deformity.

More recent studies raise some doubt about the influence of muscle imbalance, especially on hip deformity. Flexion contracture at the hip is most severe and progressive in those patients with thoracic level lesions with no motor function at the hip [2]. In these children postural factors related to greatly reduced physical activity are probably the most important factor. There was, furthermore, no evidence of spasticity in the patients with the most severe flexion contractures at the hip. Further studies [3,4] raise additional doubts about the place of muscle imbalance as the most significant cause of deformity in spina bifida.

Muscle Imbalance Due to an Upper Motor Neurone Lesion

Two-thirds of infants with myelomeningocele have an additional upper motor neurone lesion. There is an interruption of long spinal tracts with preservation of reflex activity in isolated distal segments. Reflex activity can often be mistaken

Table 4.1 Effect of the neurosegmental level of the lesion on muscle activity and limb posture

Lowest neurosegmental level functioning	Muscle acting	Limb posture
T 12		Dictated by gravity
L 1	Sartorius	Flexion/external rotation
	Iliopsoas weak	(frog position)
L 2	As above plus	
	Iliopsoas strong	Flexion and adduction at hip
	Pectineus	
	Gracilis	
	Hip adductors	
	Rectus femoris	Hip flexed and adducted
L 3	As above plus	Hip flexed and adducted
	Quadriceps	Knee extended
L 4	As above plus	Hip flexed and adducted
	Tibialis anterior (post)	Knee extended
	Medial hamstrings weak	Foot in varus
L 5	As above plus	Hip flexion
	Tensor fasciae latae	Knee in some flexion
	Gluteus medius/minim.	Foot in calcaneus
	Peroneus tertius	
	Extensor digitorum long.	
S 1	As above plus	Hip in some flexion
	Gluteus maximus	Knee in some flexion
	Biceps femoris	
	Gastrocnemius	Flattening of the sole
	Soleus	Clawing of toes
	Flexor digitorum longus	
	Flexor digitorum brevis	
	Flexor hallucis longus	
	Flexor hallucis brevis	
Lower lumbar level	With spasticity in hamstrings	Knee flexion deformity
Spastic sacral segment	With spasticity calf peronei	Foot equines
		Foot vertical talus

by parents and clinicians as useful voluntary movement. Three subtypes can be recognized.

In the first, cord function is intact down to a certain level where there is flaccid paralysis with loss of sensation and reflexes; more distally there is isolated cord function as evident from exaggerated reflex activity.

In the second the "gap" in cord function is narrow, amounting virtually to a cord transection. There is no movement of the lower limbs when the infant is crying, but a wealth of purely reflex activity (including flexion withdrawal) can be elicited by direct stimulation.

In the third subtype transection of the long tracts is incomplete and the child will have a spastic paraplegia with preservation of some voluntary movement and sensation.

Thus the muscle imbalance producing deformity in spina bifida may be of three types:

1. Normal muscle versus flaccid antagonist
2. Spastic muscle versus normal antagonist
3. Spastic muscle versus flaccid antagonist.

The last type produces the worst deformity.

There is evidence that important upper motor neurone lesions occur around the time of birth. Deformities due to spasticity are therefore not present at birth but develop in the early months of life (Fig. 4.3).

Intrauterine Posture

Sometimes deformity is present at birth in totally paralyzed lower limbs. In some of these patients the deformity may be fixed, which suggests that muscle power and imbalance have been present in fetal life. In others, the pattern of deformity suggests that it has resulted simply from pressure on paralyzed limbs.

Habitually Assumed Posture After Birth

Deformity can develop after birth in flaccid legs that are allowed to lie in one particular posture, under the influence of gravity. For example, the classic "diamond posture" or "pithed frog position" of hip flexion, abduction and external rotation in combination with knee flexion, and equinus or equinovarus at the ankle and foot.

Coexistent Congenital Malformations

Arthrogryposis

Some limb deformities resemble those seen in arthrogryposis multiplex congenita. There is rigidity and lack of normal flexion creases thought to be associated with lack of movement in utero. Such deformities are very resistant to treatment.

Traction of Nerve Roots

Some children, who have had a myelomeningocele closed at birth, may present later with progressive foot deformity (usually cavo-varus). This may be associated with spinal cord tethering which should be surgically released before correcting the foot deformity. As a result, any foot deformity which develops for the first time in the growing child should prompt a careful search for spinal cord pathology including the various manifestations of spinal dysraphism.

Fig. 4.3 The neurological lesion in spina bifida is usually asymmetrical rather than symmetrical. (**a**) The 7-year-old girl shows flexion and abduction on the left leg, adduction in the right hip. There is also spasticity in the left leg. The function of the left arm is impaired. (**b**) After correction of the flexion deformity the girl is able to stand in a hip/knee/ankle/foot orthosis

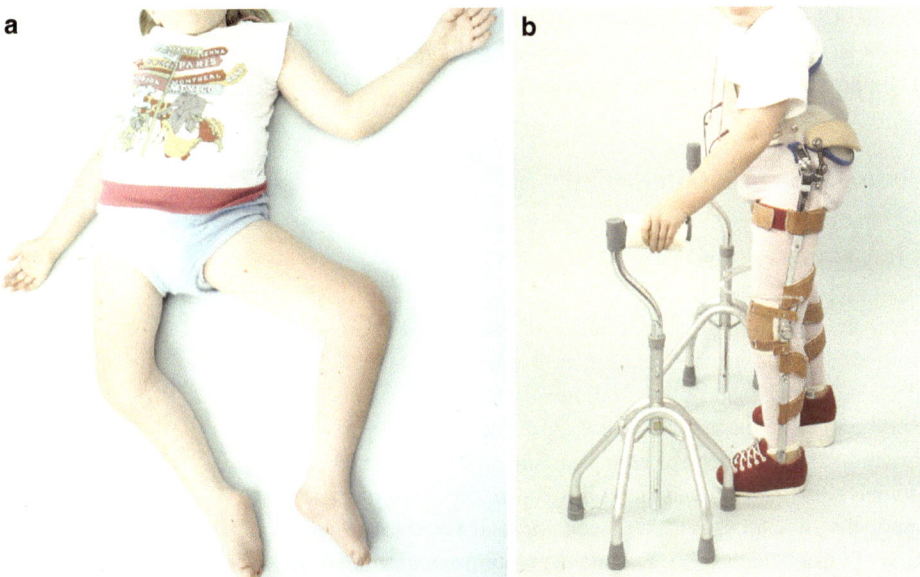

Special Risks

Pressure Sores and Chilblains

These are the result of skin insensitivity and poor circulation. If serial plasters are needed to correct deformity they should be very carefully padded because deficient pain sensation fails to warn the surgeon of pressure on the skin. In most instances, plaster casts should be used only to *maintain* the soft tissue surgical correction of deformity, not to *achieve* correction. Hip spicas should include paralyzed feet. Varus feet are always unacceptable and pressure sores inevitable. Parents should also be warned to protect their children from extremes of temperature.

Bone Fragility

Pathological fractures occur in approximately 20% of patients with paralysis in the lower limbs. Epiphyseal displacements and hyperplastic callus formation are common. Osteopenia, because of reduced muscle bulk and physical activity, is the most obvious reason for bone fragility.

Pathological fractures in patients with spina bifida are commonly mistaken for bone or joint infection (Fig. 4.4). The patient may present with a painless, red, hot, and swollen limb without a history of trauma. Radiographs will often disclose a fracture which has occurred days or weeks previously. In the later stages, if there is a delay in diagnosis and immobilization of a fracture, the florid callus may be misdiagnosed as a primary bone tumor.

The principle of treatment of pathological fractures is that immobilization of the child and the fractured limb should be kept to the minimum compatible with union in a satisfactory

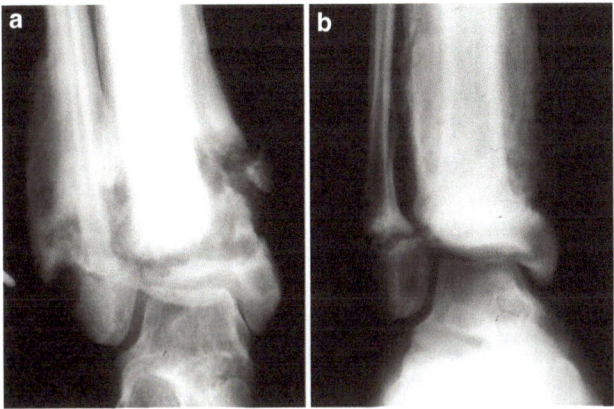

Fig. 4.4 (**a**) Pathological epiphyseal loosening of the distal tibia and fibula and exuberant callus formation in a 10-year-old girl, who did a lot of walking on her completely paralyzed feet. (**b**) After a year most of the changes have disappeared, an early closure of the growth plate must be expected

position. Well-padded hip spica casts applied with extended knees may permit early weight bearing in a standing frame, thus reducing the risk of osteopenia postoperatively [5,6]. Fractures in patients who are unable to walk can usually be adequately treated by simple closed methods avoiding invasive surgery.

Other Risks

Deficient peripheral blood flow, recurrent urinary tract infections, cognitive impairment, obesity, constipation, and respiratory problems all increase the rate of complications. So do wound dehiscence and secondary infections. Latex allergy is another potential problem: this ranges from simple contact dermatitis to bronchial edema and anaphylaxis. Care must be taken to avoid exposing spina bifida children repetitively to latex products like catheters, drips, and gloves.

Prevention and Counseling

Primary Prevention

Over the last three decades, a series of studies have demonstrated that the incidence of neural tube defects can be dramatically reduced by the administration of folic acid in very early pregnancy as neural tube closure takes place around the fourth week of gestation. Since 1998, all enriched cereals sold in the United States have been fortified with folic acid; the first time food has been fortified for the prevention of birth defects [7,8]. Despite uncertainties regarding the mechanism of action, dose, timing, and optimum method of administration, public health policy in all countries should be directed toward this simple and safe method of primary prevention of neural tube defects.

Genetic Counseling

Genetic counseling should provide the family with sufficient information on which to base a decision about further children and help them come to terms with the problems they face. Counseling should involve careful discussion of the recurrence risk for further pregnancies and the availability of antenatal diagnosis. A sympathetic understanding of the burden faced by the parents and the child and an explanation of the variability of the condition are essential.

Counseling aims to be non-directive: the family needs time to make decisions about the future. Such decisions should evolve slowly as the family learns to cope with the affected child.

Recurrence Risk

Over 90% of infants with spina bifida are born to women with no previously affected children; more than 90% have myelomeningoceles. Recurrence risk varies from area to area. Counseling should be based on local experience. The most detailed guidelines have been published in the United Kingdom. In general, the recurrence risk following the birth of an affected baby is approximately 1 chance in 25, of which half is for anencephaly and half for other neural tube defects. If the parents have had two affected children, the risk rises to approximately 1 in 10 and after three children to approximately 1 in 4. The birth of a child with anencephaly, multiple congenital vertebral anomalies, or spinal dysraphism gives

families the same predisposition to the occurrence of neural tube defects. Adult survivors with spina bifida who are contemplating a family face the same risk as the parents of a single affected child (1 in 25).

Antenatal Diagnosis

Ultrasound

Many countries offer parents screening for neural tube defects based on a maternal alpha-fetoprotein level more than twice the normal mean and associated with a risk of around 1 in 30. This indicates the need for detailed ultrasound screening. About 95% of myelomeningoceles are identifiable by the associated cranial signs which are more obvious than the spinal changes. Detection of lesions with no cranial signs is unreliable although they are likely to be less severe. Parental counseling with regard to prognosis should be guarded as although the anatomical upper level of the lesion can be estimated within one spinal level, the sensory level does not always correspond. Ultrasound at 12 weeks can virtually exclude anencephaly. Detailed morphological ultrasound can be undertaken at 18–24 weeks, but some recommend earlier transvaginal ultrasound at 14–16 weeks in severe cases although the sacrum is poorly seen before 17 weeks [9,10].

Amniocentesis

Amniocentesis for amniotic fluid alpha-fetoprotein levels and acetylcholinesterase banding is another method in addition to ultrasound but bears a risk if 1% of miscarriage from the procedure itself.

Secondary Prevention

Intrauterine diagnosis allows the abortion of babies with neural tube defects when this is acceptable to parents. Thus, antenatal diagnosis has the potential to reduce greatly the incidence of this disorder, and the recent fall in the frequency of neural tube defects in live births in England and Wales is in large part due to an effective antenatal diagnostic program.

It has been shown that there is a lower incidence of severe neurological deficit in those babies who have been delivered by caesarean section at the 36th week of pregnancy compared with those delivered vaginally at term. The parents who will not accept abortion may accept the possibility of a less severely disabled child by embracing this option. In 1998, successful fetal surgery for spina bifida was reported [11]. This approach may preserve neurological function and arrest or reverse the development of hydrocephalus and the Arnold–Chiari 2 malformation.

Prophylaxis in Subsequent Pregnancies

There is clear evidence that peri-conceptual vitamin supplementation will reduce the very high risk of a second child being affected after the birth of a child with a neural tube defect.

Coordinated Management—The Spina Bifida Clinic

A proper management program for affected children, involving as it does many disciplines and a variety of medical specialists and allied health professionals can only be properly carried out if there is a formal organization—the spina bifida clinic. The orthopaedic problems of these children cannot be managed in isolation from their numerous other problems, which should be dealt with by a minimum number of inpatient admissions and outpatient attendances by staff who have been trained in the special problems created by the condition.

The team for the clinic should include

- Coordinator
- Neurosurgeon
- Orthopaedic surgeon
- Urologist
- Psychologist and psychiatrist
- Social worker
- Physiotherapist
- Occupational therapist
- Orthotist

Adequate treatment and care of the multi-handicapped child depends upon recognizing him or her as an individual whose needs far exceed the range of the separate specialities listed above (see Chapter 3). The coordinator should be a doctor or health professional with training and expertise in managing children with multiple disabilities. The coordinator unites the clinic staff and is the person to whom parents may turn as their "general practitioner." The coordinator should possess a good working knowledge of all the specialist treatments and expertise in managing complex child and family interactions.

Such an organization offers maximum support to the family by ensuring that treatment is integrated and that attendances and admissions to hospital are properly coordinated.

Neonatal Management

The orthopaedic surgeon should examine every spina bifida child at birth or as soon as possible thereafter, not only to record basic information but to make it possible to monitor progress over the first few months and to plan orthopaedic treatment if survival seems likely. The only condition requiring orthopaedic treatment in the neonatal period is talipes equinovarus using very well-padded Ponseti serial casts (see Chapter 31) to protect the insensate skin.

Aims of Orthopaedic Management

The principal aim for those children who are thought to have the potential to stand is to establish a stable posture in extension by correcting fixed deformity. If such children are to stand for long periods and to remain on their feet in adult life, they must have their centers of gravity directly over their feet. This requires minimal flexion deformities at the hips and knees and it is ideal if there is some hyperextension at both hips and knees. About 60% of spina bifida children have neurological problems in their upper limbs and often need to use both hands for activities which other children manage with one hand. It is for this reason that we strive, where possible, to encourage them to stand for long periods without using their hands for support.

Orthopaedic surgery has different goals according to the level of the neurosegmental lesion. This level may be ill-defined because of skin lesions, other neurological deficits, or general disabilities. Furthermore, the neurosegmental level may change because of tethering of the cord. The implications of the level of the lesion with regard to walking are as follows:

- Children with thoracic lesions will not continue useful walking in adult life.
- Children with lumbar lesions may continue useful walking in adult life if they have strong quadriceps muscles and do not develop significant deformity at their hip joints. Those with strong quadriceps require not only below-knee orthoses, but may also need assistive devices (walking sticks or crutches).
- Children with sacral lesions can be expected to be useful walkers, without orthoses, into adult life. However, Bartonek et al. [12] in a 12-year follow-up study of 60 walking myelomeningocele patients at a median age of 22 years showed that 19 had deteriorated in walking ability. Important causes of this deterioration were deterioration in neurological level, development of spasticity, hip and

knee flexion deformities, low back pain, and lack of motivation. Medical problems such as strokes, sepsis, and lower limb edema were also factors.

The Functional Motor Scale (FMS) developed by Graham et al. is helpful in describing functional mobility [13]. It is meant to be uncomplicated and useful as a communication tool among health professionals. It is scored over 5, 50, and 500 m, distances thought to correlate well with mobility in the home, at school, and in the community, respectively. Dependence on walking aids is documented.

Those who will not continue walking require simple surgery to provide them with a stable posture in childhood, while those who will continue walking require more sophisticated surgery to meet the increased demands of their way of life. Because the surgery necessary in children with high lesions is relatively minor, it should if possible be performed at several levels and in both limbs under one anesthetic. Muscle imbalance must be corrected so that recurrent deformity does not occur. Radical surgery is necessary to correct rigid, arthrogryposis-like deformities especially in the feet and care must be taken to avoid pressure on insensitive skin. For this and other reasons operative correction of deformities is usually preferable to conservative methods. All management in spina bifida must involve immobilization of the child

and of the uninvolved limbs for as short a time as possible so that the incidence of pathological fractures is minimized. It should be assumed initially that all these children, except those with limited cognitive ability or gross spasticity, have the potential to stand and walk if only for a limited time in childhood. Children should be taught to stand and walk as soon as this becomes practicable. The age at which various orthopaedic procedures are recommended is shown in Table 4.2.

Gait Analysis

While the principal goal of orthopaedic surgery is to correct deformity, there are frequently secondary goals such as improving gait and function. The impact of deformity on function and gait is not always obvious. For example, the impact of hip dislocation on gait has almost certainly been overstated in previous studies and the results of tendon transfers and hip reduction are therefore frequently disappointing. Conversely, the impact of torsional abnormalities on gait has probably been underestimated. Vankoski et al. [14] demonstrated the deleterious effect of excessive external tibial torsion in myelomeningocele patients who walked with solid ankle/foot orthoses (AFOs). At the same time the beneficial effect of AFOs on gait and energy expenditure was reported [15,16].

Three-dimensional gait analysis has been used in several studies to give a good description of the typical gait patterns in children with spina bifida. Not surprisingly, kinematic deviations are closely related to neurosegmental level. Children who have sacral level lesions have a mild crouch gait with reduced power generation from the calf muscle [17]. As the neurological level ascends, greater deviations are seen because of the compensations required for increasing paralysis. At the L3/L4 level, the trunk must be moved over the stance limb to compensate for paralysis of the hip abductors and extensors, and large pelvic rotations are required to advance the limb during swing phase. Understanding these gait deviations is not just of academic interest as there are many implications for the surgical management. An abnormally wide range of hip abduction is required for independent walking in children with spina bifida. Surgery to reduce a dislocated hip, which results in stiffness, may abolish independent walking, despite a satisfactory appearance on the radiograph. A mobile lumbar spine is also a prerequisite for independent walking at the midlumbar level. Spinal instrumentation and fusion may effectively correct deformity but adversely affect gait. Three-dimensional kinematics may be used to plan reconstructive surgery and to monitor outcomes.

Table 4.2 Orthopaedic management related to stage of development and age

Developmental stage	Management
Birth	Assessment begins with a view to determine realistic aims
	Ponseti manipulation of foot deformities
First year of life Head control	Developmental stimulation
	Encourage sitting balance
Second to fourth year of life Sitting	Encourage hand skills and coordination
	Encourage upper limb strength and coordination of hand function
	Sitting aids
	Continued assessment, increased social stimulation
Upright stance	Standing orthosis
	Physiotherapy and orthoses appropriate to the neurosegmental level
	Soft tissue releases hip deformity
	Reduction of hip dislocation if indicated
	Intertrochanteric and pelvic osteotomy if indicated
Upright mobility	Tendon release or transfer in deforming foot and knee tendons
Fourth to sixth year of life	Kyphosis surgery
	Correction of fixed flexion knees
	Pelvic osteotomy in hip dysplasia
Tenth to sixteenth year of life	Correction of neurogenic scoliosis
	Correction of recurrent hip or knee deformity

Energy studies are very useful in spina bifida, explaining which gait deviations are energy expensive, identifying which children have sustainable community-walking potential, and measuring outcome after surgical or orthotic intervention [19].

Orthoses and Mobility Aids

Bracing is provided when the child shows some interest in pulling to stand. AFOs are provided at an early stage to control mobile ankle or foot deformities and provide a more stable base for standing and walking. The parapodium or a standing frame is also very useful for the younger child to introduce the experience of standing (Fig. 4.5).

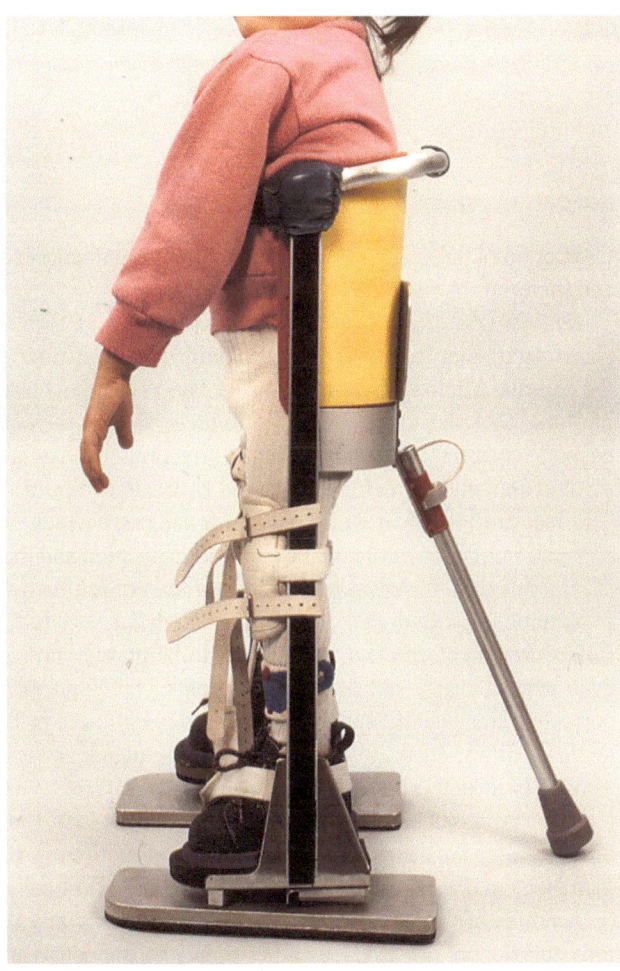

Fig. 4.5 A swivel-walker for a 3-year-old girl with high-level paraplegia to enable her stand upright

Ankle/Foot Orthosis

Floor reaction or ground reaction AFOs are ideal for the child with reasonably strong quadriceps and a paralyzed or weak calf. They provide control of the "plantar flexion–knee

extension" couple, resisting the tendency to crouch gait by promoting knee and hip extension [15] (Fig. 4.6). Rotation cables may provide additional help against the tendency of internal rotation.

Knee/Ankle/Foot Orthosis (KAFO)

A greater degree of quadriceps weakness demands that KAFOs be employed. Children will not tolerate these above-knee orthoses for long periods until they have reached an age when they no longer prefer to crawl.

Hip/Knee/Ankle/Foot Orthosis (HKAFO)

For children with more extensive paralysis, bracing is required up to hip level and a number of options are available. The parapodium is useful for the younger child, but is an aid to standing rather than walking. The swivel walker or the hip guidance orthosis (HGO) is used in some centers. Those children with some hip flexor power and no significant fixed deformity obtain great benefit from the use of the reciprocating gait orthosis (RGO) or the para-walker. The RGO is the most effective and widely used form of high bracing and offers advantages in cosmesis and acceptable energy efficiency.

Wheelchairs

Very few children in high bracing will continue with braced walking in the second decade of life. They are much more functional in wheelchairs and can attend more easily to bladder management unencumbered by high-level bracing. Children with high-level lesions and their parents should be informed at a relatively early age that a wheelchair is likely to be preferred to walking and should not be regarded as inferior to walking. Those children who have considerable paralysis, with or without gross spasticity in their legs and with or without upper limb abnormality, may never walk and will be reliant upon a wheelchair from the age of 2 years.

Children with less severe disability will commonly walk during early childhood and then, generally between the ages of 10 and 16 years, find that they are more mobile and more integrated into society, e.g., at school, in a wheelchair, and seldom stand or walk subsequently. This transition should be anticipated, planned for, and conducted after detailed discussions involving the child, the physiotherapist, orthopaedic surgeon and, in the United Kingdom, the community paediatrician (see Chapter 3). In the final analysis, the child's wishes are paramount.

Fig. 4.6 (**a**) Crouch position of both legs in a lumbar lesion with knee flexion contracture and external rotation of feet. Standing and walking is difficult for the 8-year-old boy. (**b**) Two years after surgical correction of knee flexion and foot valgus standing upright

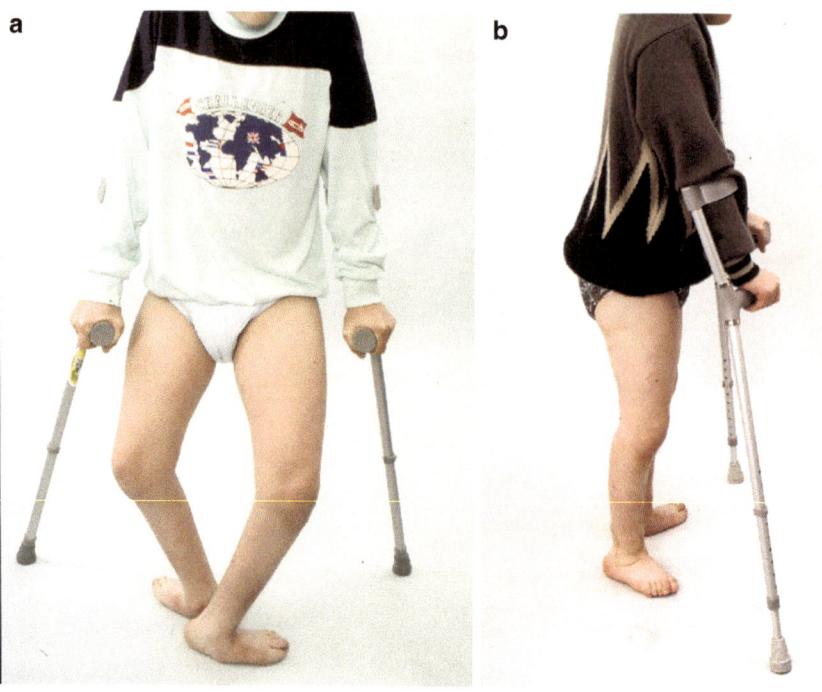

The cessation of braced walking should not be viewed as a failure but as a logical progression. It has been shown that children who have walked for a period, when compared with those who have never walked, have fewer deformities, fewer fractures, transfer more effectively, and are more mobile in the community. However, they spent longer in hospital and there were no major differences in the skills of daily living, function of the hands, and frequency and severity of obesity [19].

Management of Deformities

The Foot and Ankle

Fixed varus deformity invariably requires correction by operation, as complications from weight bearing on a small area of the sole or lateral border of the foot are otherwise inevitable. Under-correction must never be accepted since further surgery will almost certainly be required.

Valgus feet, while they remain mobile, can usually be controlled with appropriate footwear and orthoses until adolescence. Mobile valgus deformity of the subtalar joint is commonly complicated by torsional and valgus deformity of the ankle mortise: the deformity is difficult to control by bracing and surgery is often necessary to correct this complex deformity. Valgus deformity at the foot and ankle requires careful clinical and radiological evaluation including standing anteroposterior (AP) and lateral radiographs of the foot as well as a standing mortise view of the ankle (Fig. 4.7).

Correction of the valgus foot will fail if there is unrecognized and therefore untreated ankle valgus.

Equinovarus deformity. The rigidity of this deformity varies from that seen in idiopathic talipes equinovarus to the extreme rigidity of arthrogryposis. This is the most troublesome foot deformity because of its tendency to recur despite apparently adequate initial correction. Unless survival is unlikely, the deformity should be treated from birth. The feet are placed in well-padded plaster casts which are changed frequently while the baby is still in hospital and then at intervals of 4–6 weeks. More recently the Ponseti method of manipulation and cast application has been successful. Before treatment, the feet may appear to be purely varus or even calcaneovarus but as the adduction of the forefoot is corrected, it is usually apparent that there is tightness of the tendo-Achilles. In these circumstances percutaneous tenotomy is indicated. The rigid equinovarus foot will inevitably require posteromedial release (see Chapter 31) but some modifications are necessary. If the calf is not functioning, the skin incision does not need a vertical component. Portions of the tendons of the tendo-Achilles, tibialis posterior, and the long toe flexors are excised rather than just divided. Only occasionally will the degree of deformity be so mild that conservative treatment will correct the varus and adductus, leaving only equinus to be corrected by posterior release [20, 21].

Tendon transfers can play a part in children with muscular imbalance. Should the deformity recur then a repeat soft tissue release is performed. In addition a lateral wedge may be resected from the cuboid bone and fixed by K-wires.

Fig. 4.7 Paralytic talipes equinovarus. (**a**) Bilateral rigid clubfoot at 1 year of age. Manipulation and casts had failed to correct the position. (**b**) After peritalar release in both feet, satisfactory position at 2 years of age. (**c**) Both feet preserved their correction at follow-up at 12 years

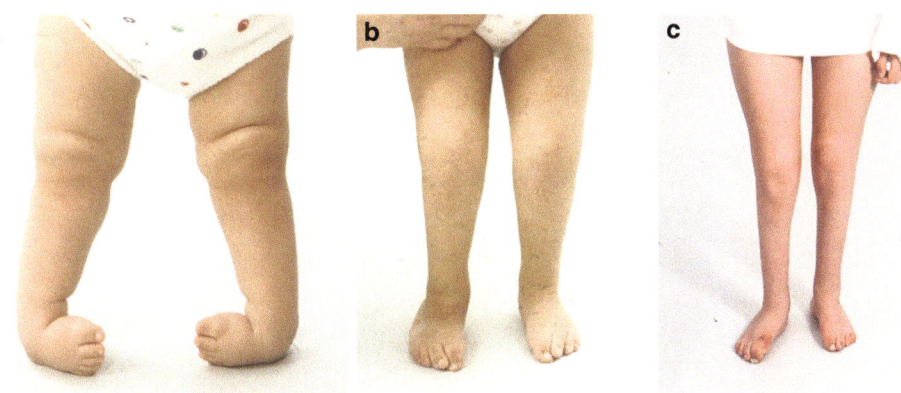

The majority of children who present with recurrent foot deformity have reduced or absent sensation. Occasionally the Ilizarov frame can help to achieve complete correction of deformity. Soft tissue releases, osteotomies, and occasionally talectomy can be used in conjunction with circular frame deformity correction (Table 4.3).

Table 4.3 Summary of talipes equino varus management in spina bifida

- Birth to 3 months: serial casting, well padded, and carefully monitored (Ponseti)
- 3–6 months: percutaneous tendo-Achilles tenotomy and serial casting
- 6–12 months: posteromedial release
- Late childhood: medial and lateral column surgery, heel and midfoot osteotomies, Ilizarov techniques
- Adolescence: heel and midfoot osteotomy

Cavus deformity. The management of this condition depends on the degree of rigidity of the deformity and the age of the child. Open division of the tight plantar structures may correct minor deformity in a young child. If the heel varus is flexible according to the Coleman block test (see Chapter 32), surgery to correct the pronated forefoot is indicated; however, if it is rigid osteotomy of the calcaneum at the age of 4 years or over is better. The efficacy of soft tissue and bony procedures may be improved by the use of an Ilizarov frame and fewer children will require salvage by triple arthrodesis at maturity.

Calcaneus deformity tends to be progressive, becomes fixed, and should be treated surgically. Transfer of the tibialis anterior to the calcaneus via the interosseous membrane is the best option. While mobile feet are preferable to stiff feet, triple arthrodesis at maturity has a useful place in the management of both varus and valgus deformity [22].

This deformity is generally left untreated until muscle power can be properly assessed at the age of 3–5 years. If the strength of the tibialis anterior is normal then this tendon is transferred through the interosseous membrane to the heel

[23]. Any other active ankle dorsiflexors are divided and, if there is fixed calcaneus deformity, an anterior ankle release is combined with this tenotomy. If the anterior muscles are spastic or if they are weak, they are divided and the tendo-Achilles is tenodesed to the fibular metaphysis [24]. The drill hole through the fibula stimulates growth at the lower end of the fibula and this may correct valgus deformity at the ankle mortise—a deformity which commonly occurs in combination with calcaneus deformity. The late-developing calcaneus deformity with a "pistol grip" heel (see Chapter 32) is best treated by osteotomy of the calcaneum, removing a wedge based posteriorly so that the tuberosity lies less vertically. At the same time restoration of muscle balance by tenodesis or tendon transfer achieves balance. More effective displacement of calcaneal osteotomies for calcaneus deformity may be achieved by using slow distraction in a circular frame.

Valgus deformity. This deformity may occur at the ankle mortise, the subtalar joint, or at both of these sites. Clinical examination and weight-bearing radiographs of the foot and ankle will clarify the site of the deformity.

Ankle valgus. Clinically the distal end of the fibula lies more proximal than the medial malleolus. Radiographs show that the lower fibular growth plate lies proximal to the ankle joint, while it should be at the same level. The lower tibial epiphysis is wedge-shaped with the medial portion of the epiphysis being wider than the lateral [25]. Under the age of 6 years this deformity may be reversed by arrest of the medial portion of the lower tibial growth plate. This arrest can be performed open using staples or by percutaneous screw hemiepiphysiodesis which is the least invasive and preferred method (Fig. 4.8).

Deformity at a later age and of a degree sufficient to present a problem should be corrected by a transverse osteotomy of the tibia with excision of a medially based wedge of lower tibia and an oblique osteotomy of the fibula. The tibial osteotomy should be approximately 1 cm proximal to the lower tibial growth plate. Any external tibial torsion that is present should be simultaneously corrected. The

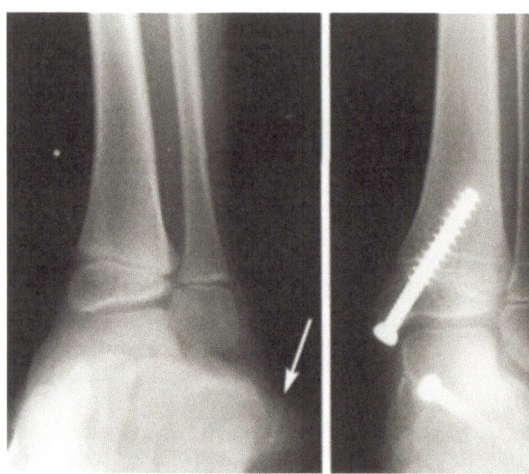

Fig. 4.8 Ankle valgus has been managed by screw epiphysiodesis through the medial malleolus and the subtalar valgus by a subtalar fusion using screw fixation and autogenous iliac crest grafting

osteotomy may be secured with a single staple or with two crossed K-wires. There is an incidence of wound breakdown and delayed union following this procedure. The Ilizarov frame is the best method of managing such complications and for revision surgery. This type of prolonged fixation, however, needs careful discussion as it is not tolerated by all children.

Subtalar valgus. If this is so gross that it cannot be controlled by an AFO under the age of 10 years then a medial

displacement calcaneal osteotomy can be performed using a threaded K-wire for fixation [26]. Calcaneal lengthening should be considered. Many prefer an extraarticular subtalar fusion in which greater correction is traded for loss of mobility [27,28]. Care should be taken not to overcorrect the deformity (Fig. 4.9).

If the patient is approaching maturity then there is commonly a plano-abductus deformity of the forefoot in association with the subtalar valgus. If the deformity is mild and easily corrigible calcaneal lengthening by the method originally described by Evans [29] and popularized by Mosca [30] may be appropriate; it needs to be combined with peroneal tendon lengthening.

Severe plano-abducto-valgus is best corrected by triple arthrodesis. The most satisfactory form of triple arthrodesis for the myelomeningocele valgus foot which generally lacks any fixed deformity but sweeps into valgus on weight bearing is the lateral inlay arthrodesis [31].

Ankle and subtalar valgus. This requires surgery at two sites. Supramalleolar osteotomy of the tibia and fibula may be combined with either calcaneal osteotomy or lateral inlay triple fusion [32] depending on the nature of the foot deformity present.

Paralytic convex pes valgus (vertical talus). This complex deformity occasionally occurs in children suffering from myelomeningocele or from diastematomyelia. The neuromuscular form of this condition is often less rigid than the classical congenital form and may develop slowly in the

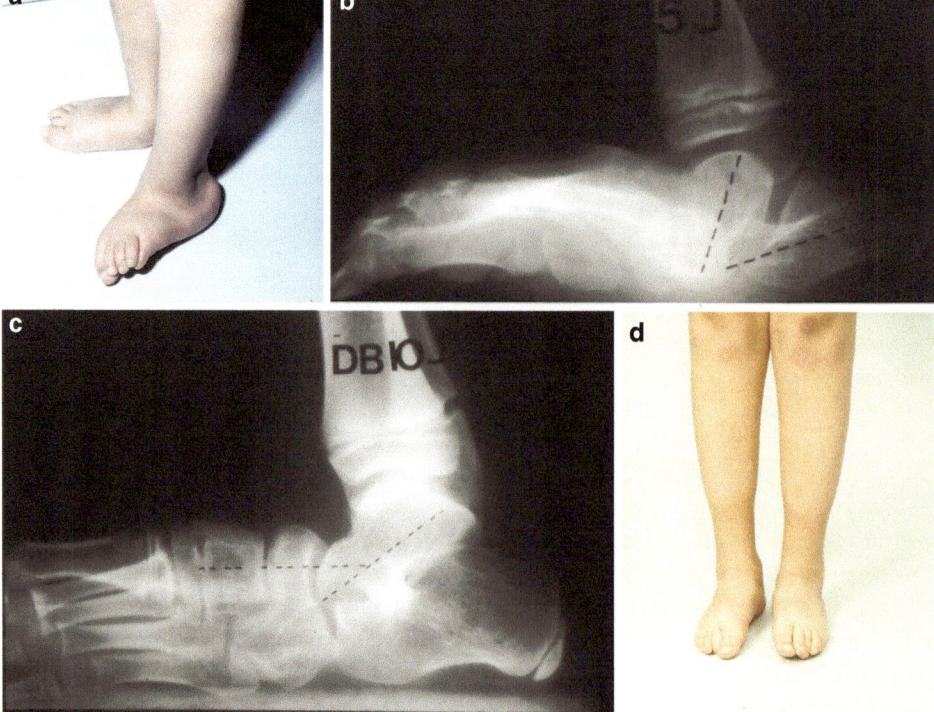

Fig. 4.9 (**a**) Rocker bottom foot in a 3-year-old girl, with problems standing on the everted foot. (**b**) Radiograph of the vertical talus. (**c**) Radiograph of the corrected foot at 10 years, 7 years after reduction of talus, and extraarticular arthrodesis after Grice. (**d**) Clinical appearance at 10 years. Full weight bearing is possible

Table 4.4 Summary of management of valgus foot

Distinguish ankle from subtalar valgus	
Young child	Ankle foot orthosis
Ankle valgus	Screw epiphysiodesis
Heel valgus—severe	Extraarticular arthrodesis (Grice); os calcis osteotomy
Heel valgus—mild	Extraarticular arthrodesis (Grice)
Abduction forefoot—mild	Os calcis lengthening
Ankle and subtalar valgus	Supramalleolar osteotomy and subtalar fusion

first years of life [33]. The management of vertical talus is described in Chapter 33.

Table 4.4 summarizes management of valgus.

The Knee

Flexion deformity and a limited range of flexion at the knee are most common in children with thoracic level lesions [3]. This suggests that muscle imbalance has been overrated as the cause of deformity in spina bifida since those with thoracic level lesions have no muscle imbalance at the knee.

The Flail Undeformed Knee

This is found in approximately 30% of those children who survive to an age at which walking may occur. Bracing is necessary to support the knees if the child is to stand and walk.

The Undeformed Knee with Quadriceps Weakness

This situation is common. Early in life bracing annoys these children because they wish to be able to crawl. Later a floor reaction orthosis may be useful. For some children a KAFO on one leg and an AFO on the other with alternate bracing on alternate days may provide an answer.

Fixed Flexion Deformity [18]

Fixed flexion deformity of up to 20° is commonly present at birth. Deformity of less than 20° can generally be ignored. If the deformity is greater than 20°, surgery in the form of a posterior release of all the hamstrings allows the child to be braced and to stand. A posterior capsular release may be needed if the tendon release fails to correct the deformity. Postoperatively the knee is immobilized in a well-padded cast enabling early standing to avoid osteoporosis as far as possible. Overzealous stretching may threaten the popliteal vessels and, if they are at risk, serial postoperative casting may be safer. Rarely, a supracondylar osteotomy of the femur is indicated (Fig. 4.10).

Limited Flexion with Recurvatum

Some neonates have a recurvatum deformity, but this usually responds to serial well-padded casting. However, the knee that is rigid in extension may have the featureless appearance seen in arthrogryposis multiplex congenita. Such knees may be treated by subcutaneous tenotomy of the ligamentum patellae. This is usually performed at the age of 6 months to

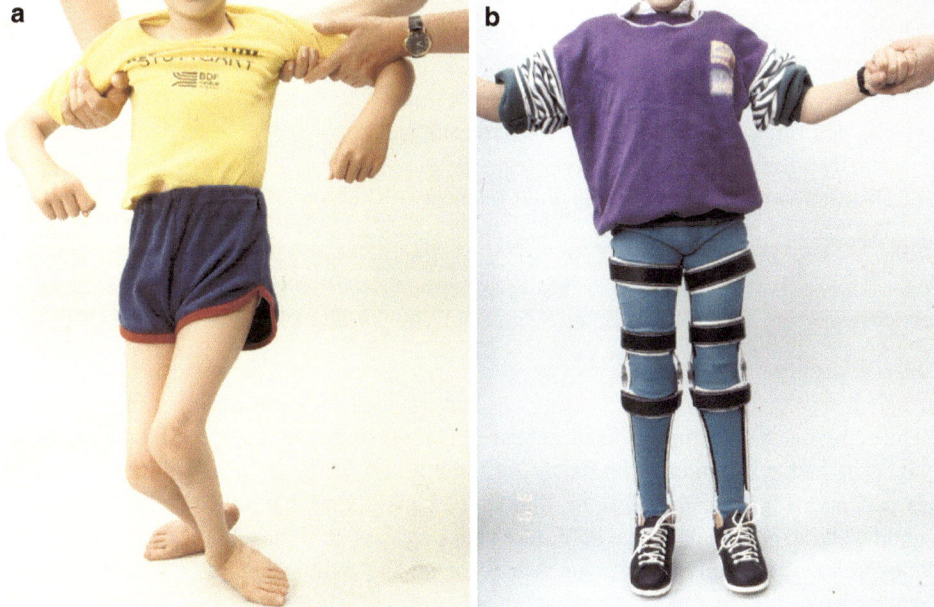

Fig. 4.10 (**a**) Flexion contractures in both knees of boy at 5 years. Inability to be braced for walking. (**b**) After tendon release of the hamstrings the boy is able to stand and walk with knee/ankle/foot orthoses

Fig. 4.11 (**a**) Fixed extension in both knees does not allow correct sitting in 3-year-old girl. (**b**) After quadriceps lengthening full flexion, good for sitting. For walking she needs knee/ankle/foot orthoses

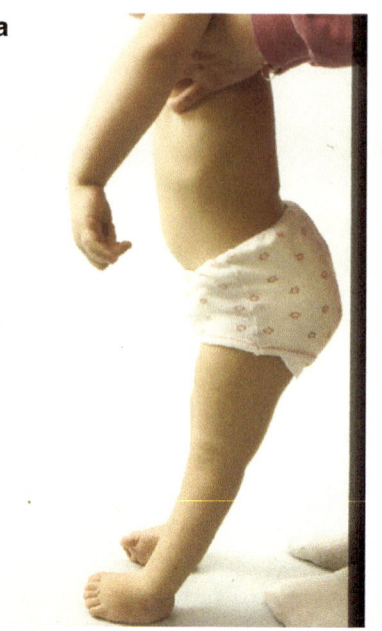
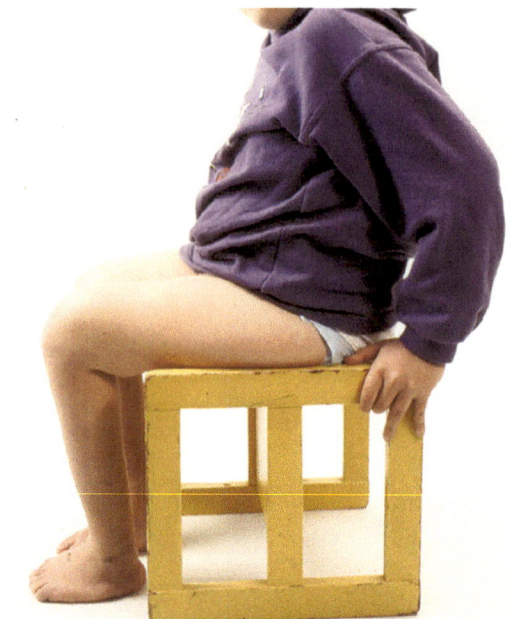

enable early crawling with flexible knees. If this is not done early at a later age when the legs are elongating they protrude when the child is seated in the classroom or a vehicle. If tenotomy is not done at an early age quadricepsplasty may be necessary (Fig. 4.11).

Valgus Deformity

This is not a common problem but may occur in children with lower thoracic or upper lumbar lesions; it may rarely require medial growth plate arrest or osteotomy.

The Hip

There are three indications to treat hip problems in spina bifida patients:

- Hip deformity which creates a problem during walking—usually a fixed flexion deformity
- Dislocation of the hip in certain circumstances
- The need to provide abductor and extensor power at the hip

Hip Deformity

The commonest deformity is fixed flexion. It is most severe and progressive in patients with flail hips [2] but is also seen in patients with lower-level lesions. Should the patient have good walking potential and the deformity is in excess of 20° and progressive, then a soft tissue release of all the tight structures in front of and lateral to the hip is performed. The

muscles are swept off both the inner and outer surfaces of the ilium, the psoas tendon is divided, sartorius and rectus femoris are released and, if necessary, the anterior capsule of the hip joint is divided transversely. At the conclusion of the procedure the anterior superior iliac spine and adjacent portions of the iliac crest will protrude anteriorly and should be trimmed.

Commonly, both hips require this procedure and both should be corrected under one anesthetic. Even if only one hip is operated upon, both should be draped to allow Thomas's test to be carried out intraoperatively. If this reveals a significant contracture, the second hip should also be released. Postoperatively the patient should be in a standing cast to prevent osteoporosis [5]. Rarely, extension osteotomy is necessary to correct gross flexion deformity in children over the age of 10 years. Proximal femoral osteotomy is a versatile procedure for the correction of multiplanar fixed deformity of the hip, using combinations of extension, varus or valgus, and derotation.

Hip Dislocation

The effect of hip dislocation on gait and function in children who have spina bifida is difficult to assess and despite many studies, the benefits of surgical reduction are difficult to define. Smith et al. [34] described and tested a questionnaire to evaluate the activities of daily living that are important to children with spina bifida and dislocated hips and their families which can be used reliably to evaluate treatment outcomes in these children.

Table 4.5 Indications for reduction of hip dislocation in spina bifida

Type of lesion	Bilateral	Unilateral
High lesions	Never	Seldom if asymmetry is no problem
Low lesions	Seldom if hip flexion contracture	Always

Reduction of the dislocated hip in spina bifida may not improve walking ability. Nevertheless some patients, particularly if the dislocation is unilateral, have a troublesome leg-length discrepancy if the hip remains dislocated. A guide to decision making is outlined in Table 4.5.

If the hip is to be reduced it is important to minimize the duration of plaster immobilization. Hip reduction should be stabilized by either Pemberton or Dega pelvic osteotomy (see Chapter 26). Six weeks only of immobilization in a standing hip spica which incorporates the feet minimizes the risk of osteoporotic fracture after operation.

Provision of Abductor and Extensor Power

The absence of functioning hip extensors and abductors at the lumbar level has been considered the main reason for hip dislocation and provides the logic for muscle and tendon transfer surgery. Sharrard [35] stressed the importance of providing abductor and extensor power and depriving the hip of the strong flexor power of the psoas muscle by performing iliopsoas transfer. It is now clear that dislocation of the hip is most common in patients with flail hips and there is doubt about the need to correct muscle balance at the hip in the prevention of hip dislocation. The iliopsoas transfer has proven advantageous in many children but has some practical and theoretical flaws [36]. Gait analysis studies suggest that the transfer continues to fire during the swing phase of gait, as a result it makes the key pelvic kinematic deviations worse and by inference it increases energy expenditure [37]. None of the tendon transfers described to stabilize the hip in spina bifida has been adequately studied objectively and the suspicion remains that they are all flawed by incorrect timing or inadequate strength. The percentage of hips reduced at follow-up is an inadequate measure of success; it is gait and function which are paramount. If a child can take steps upright but cannot climb a step the functional benefit is obviously not very good. The recurrence of flexion deformity is most often prevented by iliopsoas transfer. In addition to the posterior iliopsoas transfer (Fig. 4.12) other transfers include external oblique transfer to the greater trochanter or transfer of the adductor origin posteriorly [38].

Varus derotation osteotomy (VDRO) of the proximal femur may be used to stabilize an open or closed reduction of the hip. Given the current uncertainties regarding the value of individual operations in managing the unstable hip our current practice is pragmatic rather than scientific and based on whether there is evidence that relocating the hip will improve function and quality of life.

The unilaterally dislocated hip usually requires open reduction, psoas and adductor lengthening, Pemberton or Dega acetabuloplasty, and VDRO as a one-stage hip reconstruction. We no longer use tendon transfers (Fig. 4.13).

When there is long-standing subluxation and the acetabulum is bilocular it may not be possible to reduce the femoral head into the original acetabulum; stabilization can then be achieved by salvage, utilizing the Chiari osteotomy and/or shelf procedures.

Summary

A reducible hip subluxation is managed by VDRO. Acetabular dysplasia is managed in the younger child by a Pemberton or Dega acetabuloplasty and in the adolescent by a Chiari osteotomy or Staheli shelf.

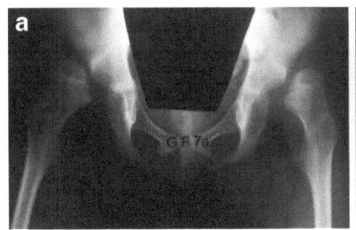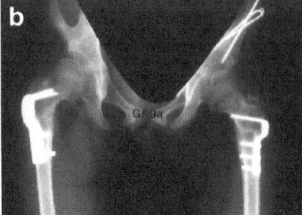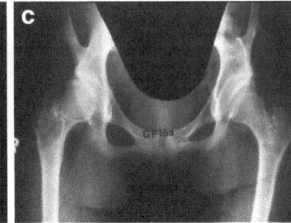

Fig. 4.12 (**a**) Bilateral hip dislocation in a 7-year-old girl, with fixed flexion and strong iliopsoas. (**b**) At 9 years after posterolateral iliopsoas transfer and reduction. After surgery the flexion contracture did not recur. (**c**) At 12 years the reduction of both hips was preserved. The girl was household-ambulatory with ankle/foot orthosis

Fig. 4.13 (**a**) Unilateral hip dislocation with asymmetry and leg-length discrepancy at 4 years. (**b**) After open reduction pelvic osteotomy and intertrochanteric osteotomy. (**c**) Pelvic radiograph at 5; 8 years symmetric hips provide equal leg length. Residual dysplasia is visible. (**d**) Symmetric standing of the patient using ankle/foot orthoses

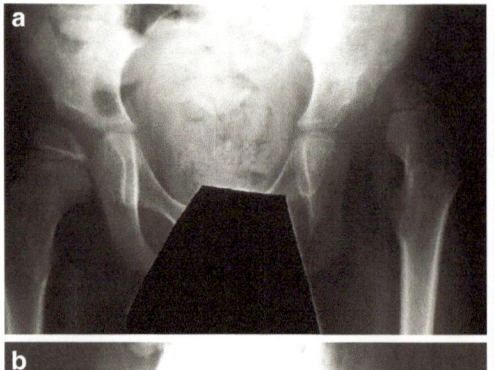

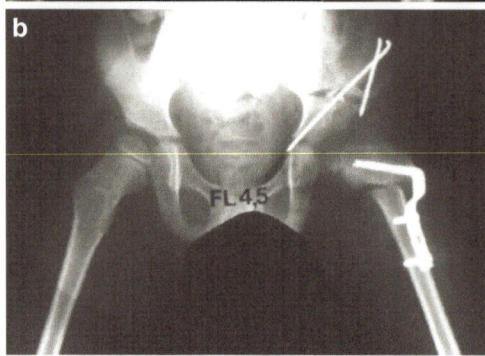

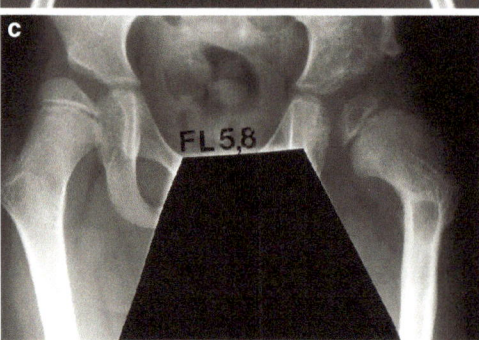

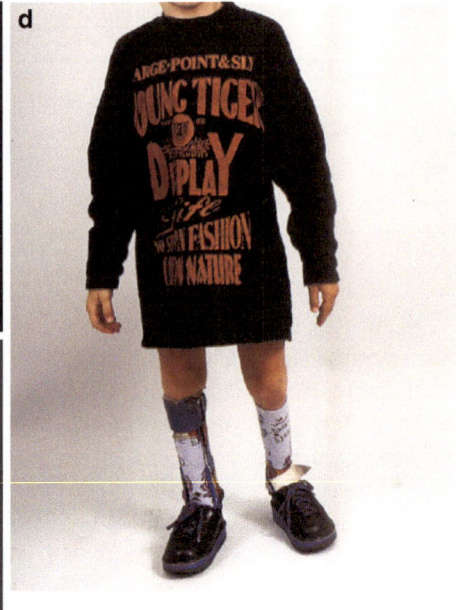

The Spine

Spinal deformity is frequently too disabling to be ignored, but conservative methods of treatment are seldom applicable.

Spinal deformity will not only impair walking but may make sitting difficult. If the child has poor sitting balance because of spinal deformity and has to use one hand to maintain upright posture, this can be a crippling impairment of function. Spina bifida patients commonly need to use both hands for functions which unaffected people can carry out with one hand because of subtle neurological disturbances in the upper limbs.

When treating the spinal deformity surgically (see Chapter 36) every effort must be made to avoid prolonged immobilization. Osteoporosis, fractures, genitourinary complications, and psychological disturbance are heavy prices to pay for a surgical complication such as infection or pseudoarthrosis. A child with spina bifida, off his feet for as little as 3 months, may never walk again.

Classification of Spinal Deformity

Spinal deformities in spina bifida patients may take one or more of the following forms:

- Defects of the neural arch and wide separation of the pedicles at the level of the neurological and meningeal lesion
- The full range of vertebral body anomalies seen in congenital scoliosis and occurring either at the level of the spina bifida or any other level of the spine. These anomalies include defects of segmentation, defects of formation, and mixed defects
- Diastematomyelia
- Spondylolisthesis
- Absence of the sacrum—partial or complete
- Kyphosis—paralytic and congenital forms
- Lordosis—commonly secondary to fixed flexion deformity of the hip and becoming fixed

- Scoliosis—the most common form of scoliosis occurring in myelomeningocele patients is paralytic in type, but congenital and mixed congenital and paralytic curves also occur. The curve may be a lordo-scoliosis or a kypho-scoliosis.

Kyphosis

Children who are born with kyphosis generally have hydrocephalus and are among the most severely affected: some do not survive. The kyphosis is generally in the lumbar spine and averages 80° at birth, increasing by an average of 8° per annum. Portions of the erector spinae muscles lie anterior to the axis of flexion and, by becoming spinal flexors, aggravate the tendency to kyphosis. Those children who are born with a lumbar kyphosis generally have complete paralysis of the leg muscles.

Management of kyphosis. The indication for correction is recurrent skin ulceration. A variety of surgical techniques are available and the choice will depend on the age of the child and the severity of the kyphosis [39,40]. A long-term review of kyphectomy in 2004 [41] reported excellent clinical results in terms of improved sitting balance and independent use of the hands despite high postoperative rates of wound healing and skin breakdown; parent and patient satisfaction levels were high (Fig. 4.14).

Procedures available include

- kyphectomy with some form of segmental posterior instrumentation and fusion
- anterior strut graft/fusion
- combinations of anterior and posterior surgery

Scoliosis

While the curve is most commonly paralytic in origin it may be congenital or mixed [42]. Furthermore, patients who have hydrosyringomyelia may develop secondary scoliosis; drainage of the syrinx may prevent progression. All children with spina bifida therefore require magnetic resonance

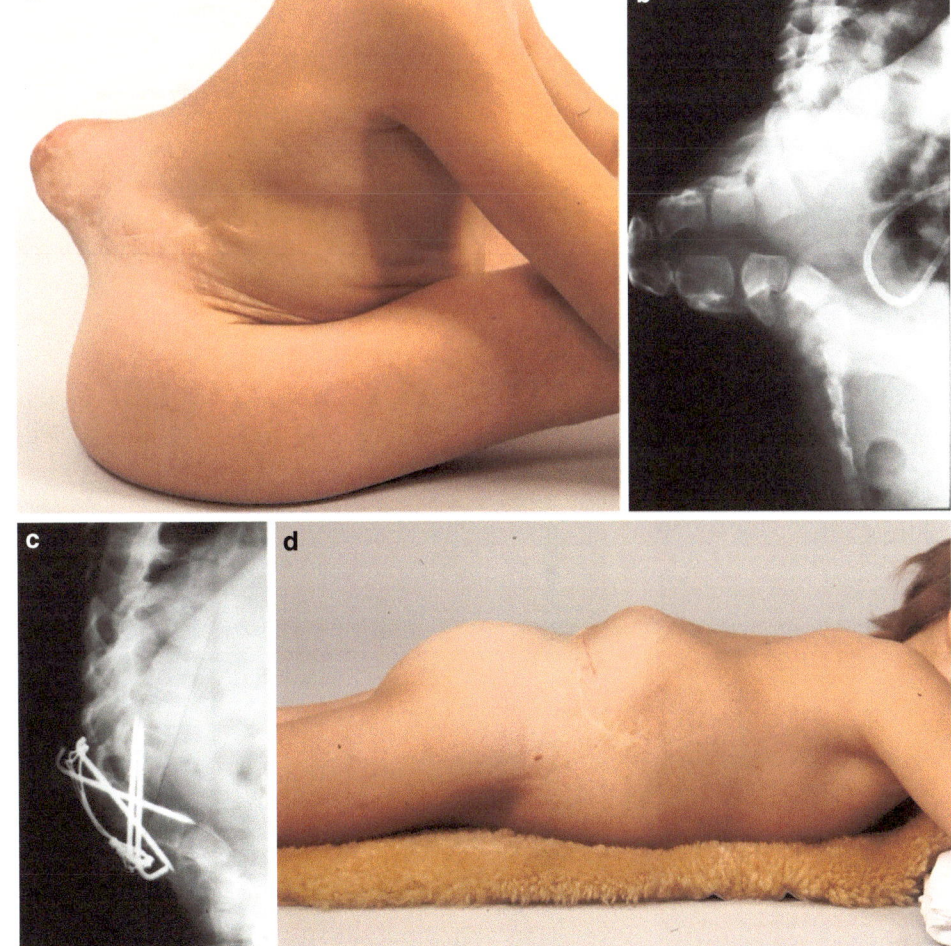

Fig. 4.14 (**a**) Fixed lumbar kyphosis in 4-year-old boy. (**b**) Radiographic view of the fixed kyphosis of 145°. (**c**) Radiographic view of the lumbar spine after excision of gibbus and tension band osteosynthesis. (**d**) Clinical appearance 2 years after surgery. There is residual kyphosis, which does not influence sitting upright and lying on the back

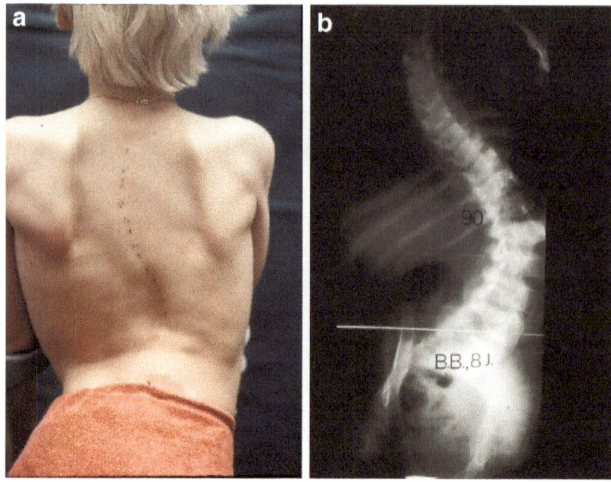

Fig. 4.15 (**a**) Severe scoliosis in a 7-year-old girl. (**b**) Radiographic appearance of the same patient shows 90° angle

imaging (MRI) of the entire cord before spinal surgery. If cord tethering is present release of the tether may help some curves smaller than 40°, but curves over 40° and thoracic curves will continue to progress [43] (Fig. 4.15).

Severe and progressive scoliosis is most common in patients with thoracic-level lesions. The incidence progressively diminishes with lesser degrees of neurological deficit.

There is a small place for bracing in children with rapidly progressive scoliosis who are considered too young for surgery.

Indications for operation include deformity increasing over 50° between the ages of 8 and 14 years, taking into consideration the child's size, the growth of the spine, and the flexibility of the curve. Less commonly other circumstances provide an indication. The main aims of surgery are

- to produce a stable fusion which will prevent further deformity;
- to provide a stable posture for standing and sitting;
- to create a level pelvis and a vertical trunk, without the need for hand support;
- to maintain maximal trunk length and remove convexities which may lead to pressure sores;
- to preserve respiratory function and satisfactory cosmesis.

The principles of surgery. Stable fusion by both anterior and posterior approaches should be considered. Anterior instrumentation enables correction of the tight curve at the apex of the primary curve (usually at the thoraco-lumbar junction) and has a high fusion rate; posterior instrumentation increases the length of spine that can be fused and allows better correction of pelvic obliquity [44] (Fig. 4.16) (see Chapter 36).

Summary

Orthopaedic management of spina bifida patients must be tailored to meet the future demands of the child. In general, those with high-level lesions and weak quadriceps muscles will place minimal demands on their feet and legs during the period when they are walking and are best served by simple surgery. This simple surgery will generally take the form of soft tissue release to free the patient from fixed deformity.

Fig. 4.16 (**a**) Ten-year-old girl with severe right convex scoliosis before correction. (**b**) Two years after anterior fusion without instrumentation followed by posterior fusion with instrumentation (with permission from Parsch D et al. [44])

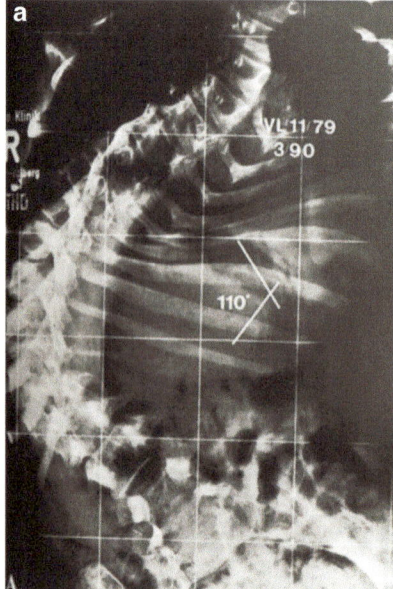
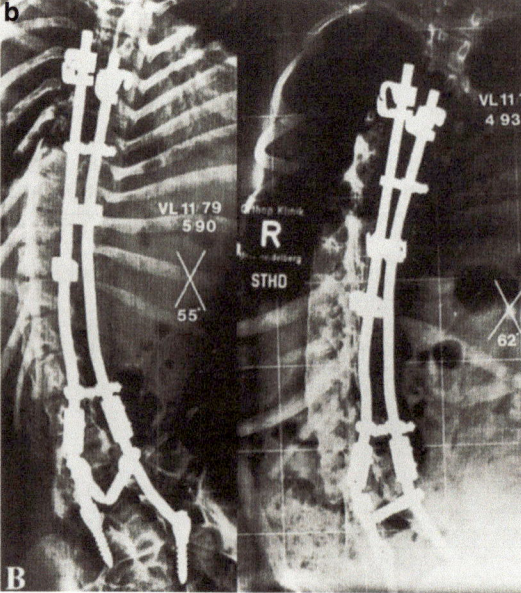

A proportion of children with low-level lesions and strong quadriceps muscles may walk throughout life or at least into adult life [12]. They put greater demands on their feet and legs [45] and benefit more from a good range of motion at the hip and knee. The role of tendon transfers to stabilize the hip and surgery for hip dislocation requires more objective study including gait analysis [46] and functional mobility scores such as that devised by Graham et al. (2004) for cerebral palsy [13] and is now being used in spina bifida patients. Plantigrade feet are essential.

Those with high-level lesions will be mobile in a wheelchair and are more likely to require radical surgery for severe spinal deformity such as scoliosis or kyphosis.

Spinal Dysraphism

This term is applied to a group of conditions in which the dorsum of the embryo forms abnormally. The condition is of importance to orthopaedic surgeons as a cause of foot deformity and leg weakness.

Definition

Spinal dysraphism refers to all forms of abnormality of formation of midline structures of the future dorsum of the embryo.

Incidence

Between 10 and 30% of the population have a degree of this abnormality be it only spina bifida occulta affecting one vertebral arch. Clinically significant spinal dysraphism is rare and the precise incidence is not known.

Embryology and Pathology

The condition may affect all or some of the primary embryonic layers to a varying degree. The type of dysplasia and the resultant conditions are illustrated in Table 4.6 [47]. Details of all aspects of the condition have been described by James and Lassman [48,49].

The commonest forms of pathology are the following:

- Diastematomyelia, where the spinal cord or filum terminale, or both, are split sagittally by a bony or fibrocartilaginous septum
- Lumbosacral lipoma

Table 4.6 Spina bifida, spinal dysraphism, or the spinal dysraphic state. Adapted from Lichtenstein (1940)

Embryonal origin	Type of dysplasia	Result condition
Cutaneous: Somatic Ectodermal	Cutaneous	Cutaneous defect Hypertrichosis Nevus Dermal sinus
Mesodermal	Vertebral	Split in spinous process Laminal defects Rachischisis
	Dural	Non-fusion of dura mater
Neural Neuroectodermal	Neural tube	Myelodysplasia Intramedullary and extramedullary growths associated with dysraphia
	Neural crest	Ectopia of spinal ganglia and of posterior nerve roots

- Meningocele manqué, in which a loop of nerve root or trunks emerges from the spinal cord, cauda equina, or filum terminale, becomes adherent to the dura, and then returns to the cauda equina or filum near to its point of origin
- Dermoid cyst
- Tight or tethered filum terminale: this may result in an abnormally distal conus (normally the conus lies at the following levels: in the fetus at the coccyx; at birth at the upper border of the third lumbar vertebra; at 5 years at the upper border of the second lumbar vertebra).
- Hydromyelia
- Atrophy meningocele
- Arachnoid cyst
- Various forms of myelodysplasia.

Frequently more than one of these abnormalities are present in combination.

Diagnosis and Differential Diagnosis

Patients may present to the orthopaedic surgeon at any age from birth to maturity. Most commonly they will present under the age of 5 years with one of the following:

- A short and often wasted leg
- A small foot
- A cavovarus foot deformity
- A paralytic valgus foot deformity
- Trophic ulceration (Fig. 4.17)

There may in addition be a cutaneous lesion in the form of a patch of hair, a nevus, a lipoma, a scarred area, or a sinus or

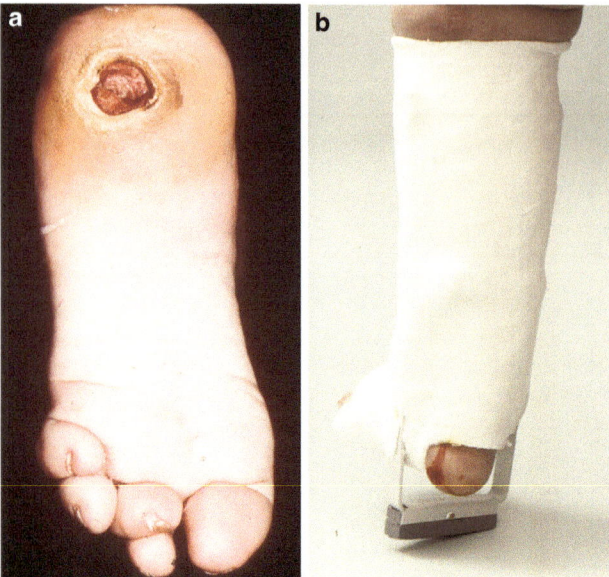

Fig. 4.17 (**a**) Perforating ulcer in a boy with spinal dysraphism with absent sensibility in this foot. (**b**) Weight relief in a walking cast and a window to take care of the trophic ulcer. The ulcer healed within 8 weeks

dimple. In a series of 200 patients [34] approximately one-quarter had no external cutaneous manifestation. Thus, it is imperative that the clinician has a high level of suspicion and carries out appropriate special investigations.

The differential diagnosis depends to some extent on the presenting features: If the child is seen with a short leg or small foot then the common differential diagnosis is hemihypertrophy or hemiatrophy. If neurological features are present then the following disorders must be excluded:

- Cerebral palsy in the form of a mild hemiplegia
- Spinal cord tumor
- Hereditary sensory and motor neuropathy
- Polyneuritis

Patients should be fully investigated, as described below, before accepting a diagnosis of "idiopathic" pes cavus (which is rarely unilateral).

Special Investigations

These will generally be performed in the following sequence (see Chapter 5):

1. *Plain radiographs.* These may disclose

   - Varying degrees and extent of spina bifida
   - A wide interpedicular distance

- Various anomalies of formation and segmentation of vertebrae
- A bony spur (if diastematomyelia is present)

It is important that the full length of the spine is radiographed in all patients.

2. *Ultrasound* (Fig. 4.15). This investigation is useful antenatally and up to the age of 6 months. Diastematomyelia is more easily identified antenatally by ultrasound than by postnatal radiographs. Both bony and cartilaginous bars can be shown [10]. Should a patient present with a cutaneous lesion on the back or a foot deformity then this investigation can clarify the nature of the underlying lesion without the need for general anesthesia.

3. *Plain computed tomography(CT)* (Fig. 4.18). *MRI* has replaced myelography. These investigations have increased the sensitivity in defining the precise nature of the spinal defect.

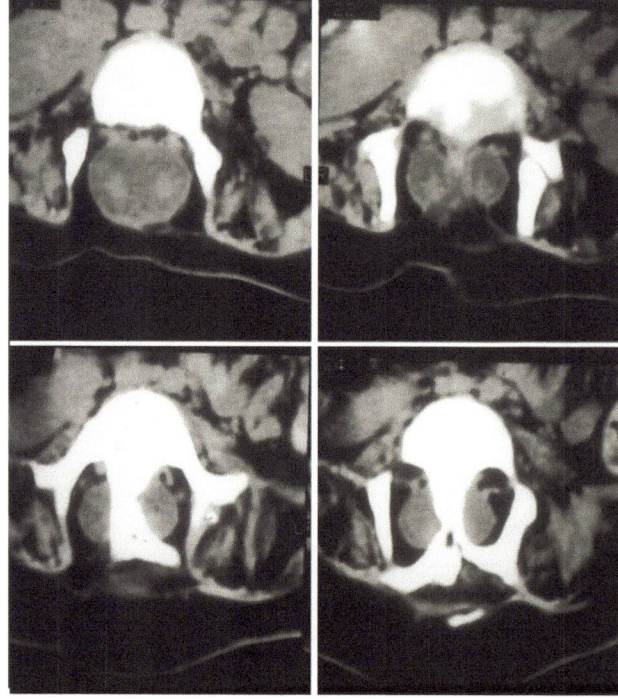

Fig. 4.18 Diastematomyelia. The CT scan of a 7-year-old girl. The spinal cord is split sagittally by a bony spur as seen on two cuts

Management of Dysraphism

The sequence of events to follow in managing a child with suspected spinal dysraphism is as follows:

1. Recognize that a neurological condition is present
2. Diagnose the cause of the condition to allow treatment of the causative spinal lesion and assessment of prognosis
3. Manage any foot deformity that is present

Recognize the Neurological Deficit

This depends on a high degree of suspicion in a child with any lower limb abnormality and in particular a foot deformity or discrepancy in foot and leg size. The clinician should look for muscle imbalance, carry out a careful neurological examination, and always examine the spine of the patient. Liaison with a paediatric neurologist is important in making a precise diagnosis and advising on appropriate investigations which should allow the neural tube defect to be accurately defined. Once clarified, the advice of a paediatric neurosurgeon should be sought.

Managing the Foot or Leg Abnormality

Cavus and other foot deformities that may be present are in general managed by

- Correcting muscle imbalance by tendon lengthening and transfer
- Soft tissue release between birth and age 5 years
- Metatarsal and calcaneal osteotomies between 5 and 10 years
- Wedge tarsectomy or triple arthrodesis at 12 years to maturity
- Circular frame correction may be used as an adjunct to conventional surgery

Complications

Deformity may recur after soft tissue releases due to persistence of the causative spinal lesion. Overzealous soft tissue release may result in reversal of the deformity.

Excessive lengthening of the tendo-Achillis may result in calcaneus deformity, which is worse than the original equinus deformity. It is generally wise to correct cavus deformity at one stage and equinus deformity at a second stage.

Postoperative casts should be carefully applied to avoid pressure on insensitive skin, particularly overlying prominent metatarsal heads.

Summary

Spinal dysraphism is one cause of abnormality in size, shape, or muscle power in the leg or foot. In the presence of such abnormalities the surgeon should always examine the lumbar spine, carry out a neurological examination, and be aware of the special investigations which are appropriate.

References

1. Shurtleff DB. Myelodysplasias and exstrophies: significance, prevention and treatment. Orlando, FL: Grune & Stratton; 1986.
2. Shurtleff DB, Menelaus MB, Staheli LT, et al. Natural history of flexion deformity of the hip in myelodysplasia. J Pediatr Orthop 1986; 16: 666–673.
3. Wright J, Menelaus MB, Shurtleff DB, et al. Natural history of knee contractures in myelocele. J Pediatr Orthop 1991; 11: 725–730.
4. Broughton NS, Menelaus MB, Cole WG, Shurtleff DB. The natural history of hip deformity in myelomeningocele. J Bone Joint Surg [B] 1993; 75: 760–763.
5. Parsch K. Origin and treatment of fractures in spina bifida. Eur J Pediatr Surg 1991; 1:298–305.
6. Dosa NP, Eckrich M, Katz DA, et al. Incidence, prevalence, and characteristics of fractures in children, adolescents, and adults with spina bifida. J Spinal Cord Med 2007; 30 Suppl 1:S5–S9.
7. Watkins ML. Efficacy of folic acid prophylaxis for the prevention of neural tube defects. Ment Retard Dev Disabil Res Rev 1998; 4: 282–290.
8. Brent RL, Oakley GP, Mattison DR. The unnecessary epidemic of folic acid-preventable spina bifida and hydrocephalus. Pediatrics 2000; 106: 825–827.
9. Broughton NS, Menelaus MB, eds. Orthopaedic Management of Spina Bifida Cystica, 3rd ed. London: WB Saunders; 1998.
10. Foster BK, Furness ME, Mulpori K. Prenatal ultrasonography in antenatal orthopaedics: a new subspecialty. J Pediatr Orthop 2002; 22: 404–409.
11. Sarwak JF. What's new in pediatric orthopaedics. J Bone Joint Surg[Am] 2003; 85A: 976–981.
12. Bartonek A, Saraste H, Samuelson L, Skoog M. Ambulation in patients with myelomeningocele: a 12 year follow up. J Pediatr Orthop 1999; 19: 202–206.
13. Graham HK, Harvey A, Rodda J, et al. The Functional Mobility Scale (FMS). J Pediatr Orthop 2004; 24: 514–520.
14. Vankoski SJ, Michaud S, Dias L. External tibial torsion and the effectiveness of the solid ankle foot orthosis. J Pediatr Orthop 2000; 20: 349–355.
15. Duffy CM, Hill AE, Cosgrove AP, et al. Three dimensional gait analysis in spina bifida. J Pediatr Orthop 1996; 16: 786–791.
16. Duffy CM, Graham HK, Cosgrove AP. The influence of ankle-foot orthoses on gait and energy expenditure in spina bifida. J Pediatr Orthop 2000; 20: 356–361.
17. Moen T, Gryfakis N, Dias L, Lenke L. Crouched gait in myelomeningocele: a comparison between the degree of knee flexion contracture in the clinical examination and during gait. J Pediatr Orthop 2005; 25: 657–663.
18. Snela S, Parsch K. Follow-up study after treatment of knee flexion contractures in spina bifida patients. J Pediatr Orthop part B 2000; 9:154–160.
19. Mazur J, Shurtleff D, Menelaus MB. Orthopaedic management of high-level spina bifida. J Bone Joint Surg [Am] 1989; 71A: 56–61.
20. de Carvalho Beto J, Dias LS, Gabrieli AP. Congenital talipes equinovarus in spina bifida: treatment and results. J Opediatr Orthop 1996; 16: 782–785.
21. Flynn JM, Herrera-Soto JA, Ramireu NF, et al. Clubfoot release in myelodysplasia. J Pediatr Orthop B 2004; 13: 259–262.
22. Olney BW, Menelaus MB. Triple arthrodesis of the foot in spina bifida patients. J Bone Joint Surg[B] 1988; 70B: 234–235.
23. Banta JV, Sutherland DH, Wyatt M. Anterior tibial transfer to the os calcis with Achilles tenodesis for calcaneal deformity in myelomeningocele. J Pediatr Orthop 1981; 1: 125–130.

24. Westin GW, Dugeman RD, Gausewitz SH. The results of tenodesis of the tendo Achilles to the fibula for paralytic pes calcaneus. J Bone Joint Surg[Am] 1988; 70A: 320–328.
25. Dias LS. Valgus deformity of the ankle: pathogenesis of fibular shortening. J Pediatr Orthop 1985; 5; 176–18.0
26. Torosian CM, Dias L. Surgical treatment of severe hindfoot valgus by displacement osteotomy of the Os calcis in children with myelomeningocele. J Pediatr Orthop 2000; 20: 226–229.
27. Gallien R, Morin F, Marquis F. Subtalar arthrodesis in children. J Pediatr Orthop 1989; 9: 59–63.
28. Bourelle S, Cottalorda J, Gautheron V, Chavier Y. Extraarticular subtalar arthrodesis. A long-term follow-up in patients with cerebral palsy. J Bone Joint Surg Br 2004; 86: 737–742.
29. Evans D. Calcaneovalgus deformity. J Bone Joint Surg[B] 1975; 57B: 270–278.
30. Mosca VS. Flexible flatfoot and skewfoot. J Bone Joint Surg[Am] 1995; 77A: 1937–1945.
31. Williams PF, Menelaus MB. Triple arthrodesis by inlay grafting: a method suitable for the undeformed or valgus foot. J Bone Joint Surg[B] 1977; 59B: 333–336.
32. Nicol RO, Menelaus MB. Correction of combined tibial torsion and valgus deformity of the foot. J Bone Joint Surg[B] 1983; 65B: 641–645.
33. Duckworth T, Smith TWD. The treatment of paralytic convex pes valgus. J Bone Joint Surg Br 1974; 56: 305–313.
34. Smith PL, Owen JL, Fehlings D, Wright JG. Measuring physical function in children with spina bifida and dislocated hips. J Pediatr Orthop 2005; 25: 273–279.
35. Sharrrard WJW. Posterior iliopsoas transplantation in the treatment of paralytic dislocation of the hip. J Bone Joint Surg[B] 1964; 46B: 426–444.
36. Parsch K, Dimeglio A. The hip in children with myelomeningocele. J Pediatr Orthop B; 1992; 1: 3–13.
37. Duffy CM, Hill AE, Cosgrove AP, et al. Energy consumption in children with spina bifida and cerebral palsy: A comparative study. Develop Med Child Neurol 1996; 38: 238–243.
38. Yngve DA, Lindseth RE. Effectiveness of muscle transfer in myelomeningocele hips measured by radiographic indices. J Pediatr Orthop 1982; 2: 121–125.
39. Fuerderer S, Eysel P, Hopf C, Heine J. Sagittal static imbalance in myelomeningocele patients: improvement in sitting ability by partial and total gibbus resection. Eur Spine J 1999; 8: 451–457.
40. Nolden MT, Sarwark JF, Vora A, Grayhack JJ. A kyphectomy technique with reduced perioperative morbidity for myelomeningocele kyphosis. Spine 2002; 15: 1807–1813.
41. Niall DM, Dowling FE, Fogarty EE, et al. Kyphectomy in children with myelomeningocele: a long term outcome study. J Pediatr Orthop 2004; 24: 37–44.
42. Guille JT, Sarwark JF, Sherk HH, Kumar SJ. Congenital and developmental deformities of the spine in children with myelomeningocele. J Am Acad Orthop Surg 2006; 14: 294–302.
43. Piez K, Banta J, Thompson J, et al. Effect of tethered cord release on scoliosis in myelomeningocele. J Pediatr Orthop 2000; 20: 362–365.
44. Parsch D, Geiger F, Brocai DR, et al. Surgical management of paralytic scoliosis in myelomeningocele. J Pediatr Orthop B 2001; 10: 10–17.
45. Duffy CM, Hill AE, Graham HK. The influence of flexed-knee gait on the energy cost of walking in children. Develop Med Child Neurol 1997; 39: 234–238.
46. Duffy CM, Hill AE, Cosgrove AP, et al. The influence of abductor weakness on gait in spina bifida. Gait Posture 1996; 4: 34–38.
47. Lichtenstein BW. Spinal dysraphism. Spina bifida and myelodysplasia. Arch Neurol Psych 1940; 44: 792–810.
48. James CCM, Lassman LP. Spinal dysraphism. Spina bifida occulta. London: Butterworths; 1972.
49. James CCM, Lassman LP. Spina bifida occulta. Orthopaedic, radiological and neurosurgical aspects. London: Academic Press/New York: Grune & Stratton; 1981.

Chapter 5

Poliomyelitis

Wang Chow, Yun Hoi Li, and Chi Yan John Leong

Introduction

Poliomyelitis is a highly infectious viral disease that mainly affects young children. It spreads through contaminated food and water. The virus may attack the central nervous system and cause paralysis and subsequent deformity. The first known description of poliomyelitis was given by Underwood in 1789 and it was not until 1855 that Duchenne described the pathological process in poliomyelitis involving the anterior horn cells of the spinal cord.

The disease had been endemic worldwide before the introduction of an effective vaccine and the launch of a global vaccination program. In 1988, the Global Polio Eradication Initiative was launched by the World Health Organization (WHO), Rotary International, the US Centers for Disease Control and Prevention (CDC), and UNICEF. The number of cases has fallen by 99% from an estimate of more than 350,000 cases in 1988 to only 1951 reported cases in 2005. The disease was widely endemic on five continents in 1988 and is now found only in parts of Africa and south Asia. At the time of writing, there are four countries, Nigeria, India, Pakistan, and Afghanistan with endemic polio, down from more than 125 countries in 1988 [1–3].

Etiology and Immunization

The disease is caused by one of the three types of poliomyelitis virus (Brunhilde, Lansing, and Leon) belonging to the enterovirus group, which includes Coxsackie C and the ECHO viruses. The last two viruses can produce a clinical picture indistinguishable from that of poliomyelitis. The lack of cross-immunity between each type of polio virus makes reinfection possible.

W. Chow (✉)
Department of Orthopaedics and Traumatology, Hong Kong, China

The virus is most commonly transmitted through the gastrointestinal tract from infected food or fecal matter, although the disease may also be contracted via the respiratory tract. The virus is blood-borne to the central nervous system. Epidemics used to occur during summer and autumn; however, with the widespread use of oral vaccine, epidemics are now unusual.

Two types of vaccines are available. The Salk vaccine, first introduced in 1954, is a killed vaccine given by injection, whereas the Sabin vaccine is a live, attenuated oral vaccine [4]. The latter type is cheaper, safer, and more effective against all three types of polio virus. Immunity conferred is usually lifelong. However, recent attention has been given to the vaccine-associated poliomyelitis caused by the oral vaccine. The risk of contracting poliomyelitis from the vaccine is extremely low, with a rate of 1 case per 2.5 million doses. The CDC has reported complete elimination of this vaccine-associated poliomyelitis in 2006 after a change of vaccination program. The child is now first inoculated with the inactivated vaccine, followed by the oral attenuated one.

Pathology

Acute Stage

Poliomyelitis starts as a systemic infection. The incubation period varies from 1 to 3 weeks. Initial extraneural involvement is mainly in the reticulo-endothelial system, with hyperplasia of the spleen and lymph nodes. Only 1–2% of those affected ultimately suffer from neural damage.

Neural involvement occurs chiefly in the brain stem and anterior horn cells of the spinal cord. However, inflammatory changes may occur in the posterior ganglia and nerve roots.

Initially, the spinal cord shows inflammatory changes, with polymorphonuclear cell infiltration, later replaced by lymphocytes. There are varying degrees of neuronal degeneration, with cell death and disintegration being the worst histological signs after a few days. Glial cell replacement occurs as the chronic stage of the disease appears. Because of anterior horn cell involvement, there is lower motor neurone paralysis, especially of muscles innervated by the cervical and lumbar enlargements. Flaccid paralysis is present, with normal sensation in the extremities. Intramuscular injection during the acute stage may lead to localization of paralysis in a certain segment of the cord. Similarly, surgery such as tonsillectomy may trigger the appearance of bulbar palsy.

Chronic Stage

Residual paralysis is of varying severity and combinations. The muscles of the lower limb are affected at least four to five times more often than those of the upper limb. The quadriceps, glutei, tibialis anterior, hamstrings, and hip flexors are involved, in descending order of frequency. The intrinsic muscles of the foot are sometimes affected. In the upper limb, the deltoid, triceps, and pectoralis muscles are commonly affected. Trunk muscles are weakened less often.

After the initial stage of muscle irritability and spasm, atrophy and fibrosis set in. Muscle imbalance leads to joint deformity and sometimes dislocation. This is often aggravated by gravity, posture, and subsequent growth of the child. Secondary contracture of the tendons, ligaments, joint capsule, and sometimes the skin, all add to the rigidity of the deformity. Because paralysis occurs in a growing limb, shortening will develop. The bones are thin and sometimes osteoporotic and prone to fracture. The joints may show restricted mobility with possible subluxation or dislocation. Osteoarthritis does not commonly occur unless there has been previous operation or trauma.

The respiratory system may be affected secondary to bulbar palsy or paralysis of the ventilatory muscles (intercostals or diaphragm). Bulbar palsy usually recovers fully.

Recovery Prognosis

Most functional recovery in muscle power occurs within the first few months and is complete by 6 months after the initial illness; theoretically, recovery is possible for up to 2 years. Good prognostic factors for recovery include young age, partial paralysis, and upper extremity involvement. Careful muscle charting, followed by serial assessment during the initial few months, is therefore important as a means of assessing the likelihood of recovery.

Clinical Features

Acute Stage

Acute symptoms include fever and malaise. Symptoms of encephalomyelitis appear within a week: severe headache, vomiting, neck rigidity, meningism, and backache are common. Simultaneously, paralysis of the extremities occurs. Asymmetrical involvement of the lower extremities is the most common pattern. Absence of progression of muscle paralysis heralds the end of the acute phase. Signs during the early stage include muscle spasm, with tenderness on palpation. With impending paralysis of the affected limb, the deep tendon reflex is either exaggerated or decreased. The superficial reflexes are usually absent initially. Irritation may be present, but sensation of the limb is normal.

Upper limb muscle paralysis affects the shoulder girdle more often than the arm. Particular attention must be paid to detecting paralysis of the intercostals and diaphragm. Neck muscle weakness may be associated with difficulty in swallowing. Lower limb muscle paralysis is invariably associated with back and abdominal muscle weakness and the quadriceps are most frequently involved [5]. The acute stage usually lasts 1–2 weeks.

Convalescent Stage

This is the stage in which muscle recovery occurs. It lasts for 2 years after the acute illness. Serial muscle charting is necessary, especially in the first few months, when most of the recovery is expected. Initial examination may be difficult because of muscle pain or spasm. Loss of recovery potential in some muscles may occur if excessive activity is allowed in the early convalescent stage. Contractures of fascia, muscle aponeurosis, and muscle itself begin during this period.

Chronic Stage

No muscle recovery is expected 2 years after the onset of the disease. By then, the orthopaedic surgeon is best placed to utilize residual motor activity. Deformities may be fixed or mobile: with time, some mobile deformities, if neglected, can become fixed. Growth and posture further aggravate the joint deformities. Initially, only the soft tissues are involved, but later secondary changes occur in bone and joint. The younger the patient, the greater the chance of significant deformity [6, 7]. Common deformities in the chronic phase are shown in Table 5.1.

Table 5.1 Common deformities in the chronic phase of poliomyelitis

Site	Lesion	Effect
Upper Limb		
Shoulder	Deltoid paralysis	Weakness of shoulder abduction
Elbow	Flexor paralysis	Inability to flex the elbow
Forearm	Fixed supination	Inability to pronate interfering with the position of the hand in daily activities
Wrist	Extensor weakness	Inability to dorsiflex the wrist
Hand	Intrinsic paralysis	Impaired hand function
Thumb	Thenar muscle loss	Lack of opposition of the thumb
Lower limb		
Hip	Relative overaction of the hip flexors and adductors	Paralytic dislocation
	Contracture of anterior and sometimes lateral structures	Flexion or flexion–abduction contracture
	Gluteal paralysis	Usually mixed extension–abduction weakness
	Extensive weakness of muscles around hip	Flail hip
Knee	Strong hamstrings and weak quadriceps	Flexion contracture
	Contracted ilio-tibial tract	Genu valgum and external tibial torsion
	Weak quadriceps and lax soft tissue at the back of knee	Genu recurvatum
	Extensive paralysis around the knee	Flail knee
Foot and ankle	Weak tibialis anterior and weak tibialis posterior	Equinovalgus contracture
	Weak tibialis posterior only (rare)	Eversion deformity
	Weak tibialis anterior, peronei, and toe extensors	Equinovarus deformity
	Weak triceps surae	Calcaneus deformity
	Overactive long toe extensors (with weak ankle dorsiflexors)	Claw toes
	Overactive long toe flexors (with weak triceps surae)	Pes cavus and calcaneus
	Imbalance between intrinsic and extrinsic foot muscles	Pes cavus
	Shortened muscles affect bone growth	Leg length discrepancy
Trunk		
Spine	Asymmetric paralysis of paraspinal muscles. Ilio-tibial tract contracture and pelvic obliquity	Scoliosis
	Ilio-tibial tract contracture (hip abductor contracture)	Pelvic obliquity
	Leg length discrepancy	
	Scoliosis	
	Weak abdominal muscles	

Diagnosis

The diagnosis of poliomyelitis is largely a clinical one. The prodromal phase is similar to other viral infections of the gastrointestinal or upper respiratory tracts. It may pass unnoticed, especially if it is not followed by neurological problems. The poliomyelitis virus may be found in the throat swab or stool. The diagnosis is usually made at the paralytic stage (see differential diagnosis below). Laboratory investigation shows nonspecific changes, such as a slight increase in the erythrocyte sedimentation rate and a leucocytosis. Lumbar puncture yields clear, pus-free fluid.

There may be an increase in cerebrospinal fluid pressure, together with an increase in the white blood cell count, initially neutrophils, but later lymphocytes. The protein content in the cerebrospinal fluid may increase. Attempts at culture of the poliomyelitis virus from the cerebrospinal fluid are rarely useful, and other sophisticated laboratory tests are impractical. Patients in the chronic stage cease to reveal these changes.

Differential Diagnosis

Acute Stage

- Any cause of meningitis or encephalitis
- Guillain–Barré polyneuritis
- Bone and joint infections
- Pseudoparalysis of whatever cause
- Myalgia or acute paraplegia of whatever cause
- Acute rheumatic fever

Chronic Stage

- Tuberculosis/spinal infection
- Transverse myelitis
- Spinal/spinal cord tumor
- Cerebral palsy
- Talipes equinovarus

Management

General

During the acute stage, the patient is usually under the care of a paediatrician. General, supportive treatment is necessary. Ventilatory failure requires active resuscitation and the prevention of complications. Tracheotomy, assisted ventilation, chest physiotherapy, and antibiotics may be needed, particularly for patients with bulbar involvement who need expert ventilatory monitoring. Bed rest and fluid replacement are necessary, but sedatives should be avoided because they cause further depressant effects.

The orthopaedic surgeon should be involved even in the acute stage. Muscle spasm is relieved by hot packs and contractures are prevented by early splintage of the joints in a functional position. Particular attention should be paid to prevent equinus contracture of the ankles by well-padded ankle–foot splints and deformity of the knees by support with a small roll behind the knees. The hips are protected by keeping the thighs in slight abduction and neutral rotation and the deltoids by holding the arms in mild abduction and neutral rotation. Physiotherapy should be started gently (especially while the irritable stage is subsiding), consisting of gradual gentle stretching of spastic muscles by passively putting the joints through the normal range of motion. In the later stage of the acute phase, assisted muscle exercises lead gradually to an active exercise program.

Management of Established Contractures

Basic Principles

Secondary factors frequently worsen the effects of a primary muscle imbalance, producing fixed contractures. These secondary factors consist of contractures of the joint capsule, aponeurosis, neurovascular bundle, and skin, and deformity of joint surfaces.

Gentle stretching of a joint contracture is very useful, but care must be exercised during manipulation because the osteoporotic bone is prone to fracture or the epiphysis may slip. When the contracture has been fully stretched, the joint is splinted in an overcorrected position but removed from the splint for mobilization every day.

Dynamic splintage is preferred to static splintage. If conservative treatment fails, consideration should be given to surgical correction. The following clinical factors must be taken into account:

- The degree of contracture in the adjacent joints of the ipsilateral limb
- The status of the contralateral limb
- Residual power of the lower limbs as a predictor of independent walking, with or without calipers
- Residual power of the upper limbs (especially triceps function, to enable the patient to use elbow crutches)

As a general rule, older patients with severe deformities respond poorly, but young patients with mild to moderate fixed deformity are suitable candidates for surgery.

Provision of motor power after correction of contractures is important in management. This requires the application of the basic principles of tendon surgery [8], sometimes in combination with bony stabilization procedures (preferably delayed until bone maturity).

Orthotic splintage is necessary not only to keep the manipulated joint in the overcorrected position to prevent recurrence of deformity but also to augment weak muscles and to protect paralyzed muscles from overstretching. Tendon transfers should also be protected from overstretching in the first few months after surgery.

Upper Limbs

Shoulder

The most common upper limb muscle that is paralyzed in poliomyelitis is the deltoid, followed by the elbow flexors and extensors. In the hand, the opponens pollicis is the most often involved [9]. Reconstructive procedures for the shoulder are not indicated unless there is good function of the arm, forearm, and hand [10].

Deltoid Paralysis

The deltoid and the clavicular head of the pectoralis major are the two prime movers of the shoulder joint. Paralysis of the deltoid results in the loss of abduction power. Deltoid paralysis is usually partial, with sparing of the posterior portion, and therefore transfer of trapezius is recommended [11]. However, multiple muscle transplantation in stages may be necessary (depending upon the remaining muscle power) using the clavicular fibers of pectoralis major, the remaining posterior portion of deltoid, the origin of the long head of triceps and the short head of biceps, latissimus dorsi, and teres major [12–15]. The possible transfers are detailed in Table 5.2.

Shoulder Arthrodesis

Extensive muscle paralysis around the shoulder causes subluxation or dislocation. When this becomes symptomatic, shoulder arthrodesis may be considered, provided that

- good scapulothoracic control by trapezius and serratus anterior compensates for the loss of glenohumeral movement
- the limb functions well distal to the shoulder

The exact position of shoulder arthrodesis is controversial; the position should allow the hand to reach the face for feeding and cleaning and the perineum for toileting.

Table 5.2 Possible substitute by transfer

Muscle paralyzed	Substitution
Subscapularis	Superior portion of serratus anterior
Supraspinatus	Levator scapulae or sterno-cleidomastoid
Subscapularis/infraspinatus	Latissimus dorsi or teres major
Serratus anterior paralysis	Pectoralis minor by posterior transfer

Excellent results are generally seen in patients with good elbow and hand function [12, 16–18]. The recommended position for children is 45° of abduction, 25° of flexion, and 25° of internal rotation [19]. Rowe recommended fusion in 20° of abduction, 30° of flexion, and 40° of internal rotation for adults. Major disability in any patient who has had an arthrodesis of the shoulder is related to the lack of internal rotation as it is important for the arm to reach the midline [20]. The angle of abduction should be determined by the angle between the shaft of humerus and the vertebral border of the scapula instead of the angle between the arm and the lateral thoracic wall.

Elbow

Flexor Paralysis

Loss of elbow flexion power is very disabling because the patient cannot bring the hand to the head and mouth. Treatment of elbow flexor paralysis is indicated only if the patient has good hand function. The spread of neurological involvement of the whole upper limb and the associated functional loss should be assessed in detail before planning any surgery. Reconstruction of the hand should precede procedures at the elbow. Weakness of the muscles around the shoulder and wrist are contraindications to reconstruction.

The most commonly used substitute for the elbow flexors is the wrist flexor mass (Steindler's flexorplasty) [21], in which the medial epicondyle and the origin of the wrist flexors are transferred proximally to the lower humerus. Possible complications include the development of a fixed pronation deformity and a mild flexion contracture of the elbow. Failure of the operation may be due to initially weak wrist flexors or poor fixation of the medial epicondyle to the humerus. A posterior bone block operation may prevent a weak elbow flexor from becoming overstretched.

When Steindler's flexorplasty is not feasible, other muscle transfers may be considered to reconstitute elbow flexion. The muscles that have been used include the whole group of pectoralis major (Brooks–Seddon procedure), sternal head of pectoralis major (Clark's procedure), latissimus dorsi (Hovnanian procedure), and triceps (Table 5.3) [22, 23].

Triceps Paralysis

Gravity assists elbow extension and thus partly compensates for loss of triceps function. However, when active, forceful elbow extension is needed, as in crutch walking or transferring from bed, strong extension is needed. Possible transfers include brachio-radialis or latissimus dorsi. The latissimus dorsi has a long neurovascular bundle, making mobilization of the muscle easy.

Table 5.3 Transfers to produce elbow flexion

Muscle transfer	Comment
All of pectoralis major muscle (Brooks–Seddon procedure)	Clavicular portion of pectoralis major must be strong. Used when the biceps brachii is completely paralyzed. Muscle control of shoulder and scapula must be good
Sternal head of pectoralis major (Clark's procedure)	Used when the clavicular portion of pectoralis major is paralyzed
Pectoralis minor	Used when pectoralis major and biceps are paralyzed. A fascia lata graft is necessary to bridge the gap
Sterno-clavicular head of sterno-cleidomastoid muscle	Fascia lata graft to bridge the gap; may cause webbing of the neck
Latissimus dorsi muscle (Hovnanian procedure)	Provides good cross-sectional area and strength for the transfer. Origin of latissimus dorsi transplanted into biceps tendon
Triceps anterior transfer	Indicated when other transfers are not feasible. Active extension of the elbow may be weakened

Forearm

Pronator Contracture

Supination is restored by transferring pronator teres and flexor carpi radialis around the ulnar border and the dorsum of the forearm to the radio-volar aspect of the radius.

Supinator Contracture

This is usually associated with a strong biceps. When there is insufficient power for tendon transfer, osteotomy of both forearm bones and stabilization in an overcorrected position are necessary. The alternatives for fixed deformity include interosseous membrane release, release of the radio-ulnar joints, and biceps lengthening.

Wrist

Wrist drop develops if the wrist dorsiflexors are involved; it can be controlled by a splint. If this improves finger function, a wrist arthrodesis may be indicated.

Fingers

Clawing of the fingers is the result of intrinsic muscle paralysis. The thumb lacks active opposition because of involvement of opponens and the short abductor muscles. The classical Bunnell transfer is sometimes helpful in providing opposition, but the flexor digitorum sublimis that is to be transferred from the middle or ring finger must have at least Medical Research Council (MRC) grade 4 power. The remaining profundus muscle must be strong enough to flex the finger [24, 25].

Lower Limbs

The aim of surgery in the lower limb is to provide a stable, balanced gait, with or without a caliper. Muscle contracture and imbalance, contracture of intermuscular septa and fasciae, shortened tendons, and retardation of bone growth all contribute to difficulty in walking. The patient presents with an abnormal gait. Examination of the lower extremities should concentrate on the presence and extent of fixed or mobile deformity, the range of motion of the joints, residual muscle power, leg length discrepancy (both real and apparent), and concomitant pelvic obliquity. Lower limb deformities are usually multiple, so good initial documentation is necessary, followed by careful planning. In general, the hip problems, usually a contracture, should be dealt with first. Sometimes, deformities can inhibit a weakened muscle, and release of such deformities places the weakened muscle in a mechanically more advantageous position [26–28].

Hip

Flexion or Flexion–Abduction Contracture

The offending structure is usually a contracted ilio-tibial tract and lateral intermuscular septum. This tether is very often associated with an anterior soft tissue contracture (rectus femoris, tensor fasciae latae, sartorius, ilio-psoas, and the

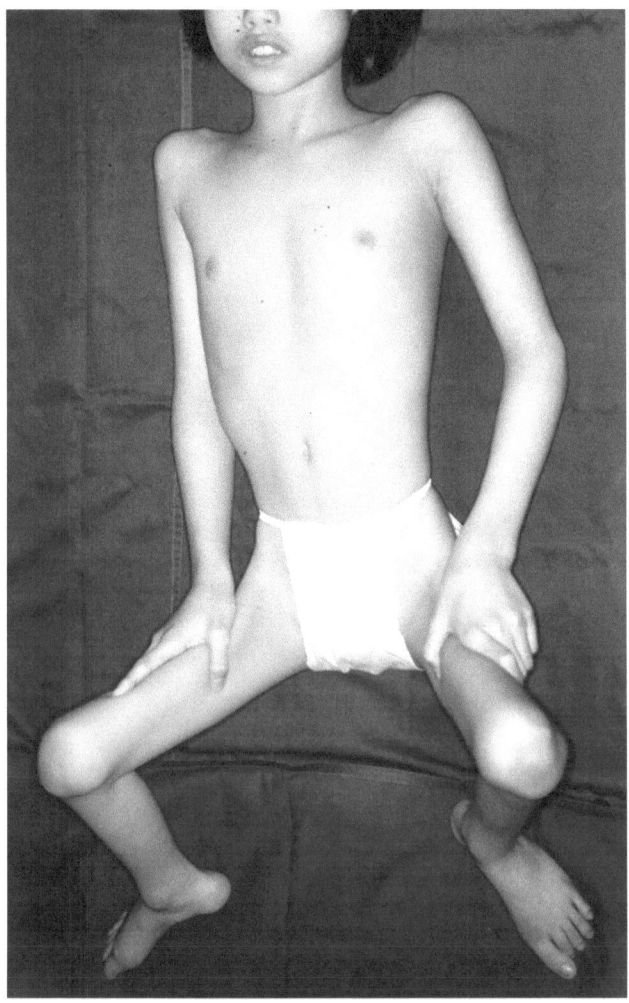

Fig. 5.1 A patient with flexion–abduction contractures of both hips

hip capsule), further aggravated by weakness of hip extension (gluteus maximus) and hip abduction (gluteus medius) (Fig. 5.1).

The ilio-tibial tract lies anterior to the hip and posterior to the knee joint and therefore produces a flexion contracture of the hip and knee. The Ober test is performed to elicit an abduction contracture [29]. The patient lies on his normal side, with the thigh on the examination couch and the hip and knee flexed enough to obliterate any lumbar lordosis. The knee of the affected leg is flexed to a right angle and the hip initially in a flexed position. The examiner grasps the ankle lightly with one hand and steadies the patient's pelvis with the other. The affected leg is extended so that the thigh is in line with the body. If there is any abduction contracture, the leg will move into abduction. This tight band can be easily felt with the examining fingers between the crest of the ilium and the anterior aspect of the trochanter. The Ober test can be modified by putting the patient in the prone position; the amount of hip abduction tightness can be assessed

with hip extended and knee flexed. This method reduces the movement of the pelvis that may occur when the patient is lying on his side [30].

Unilateral or asymmetrical abduction contracture will produce a pelvic obliquity and lumbosacral scoliosis and the contralateral hip is prone to subluxate. In addition to this, a contracted ilio-tibial tract will also produce a flexion and valgus deformity of the knee joint in association with external tibial torsion (Fig. 5.2) [31, 32]. In severe cases, posterolateral subluxation of the knee joint may occur. Another sequel of the external tibial torsion is the compensatory varus deformity of the foot which will disappear after the tibial torsion is corrected [33]. If the soft tissue contractures and muscle imbalance are not treated, further secondary bony deformities will progress with growth.

Surgical release of anterior soft tissue contracture can be achieved proximally with Ober's fasciotomy and distally with Yount's procedure [29, 34]. In mild cases, distal release with sectioning of the ilio-tibial tract together with a portion of the lateral intermuscular septum alone is simple and effective. If adequate correction cannot be obtained with the distal release in more severe contracture, Ober's procedure can be performed at the same time. The contracted muscles that must be released include tensor fasciae latae, gluteus

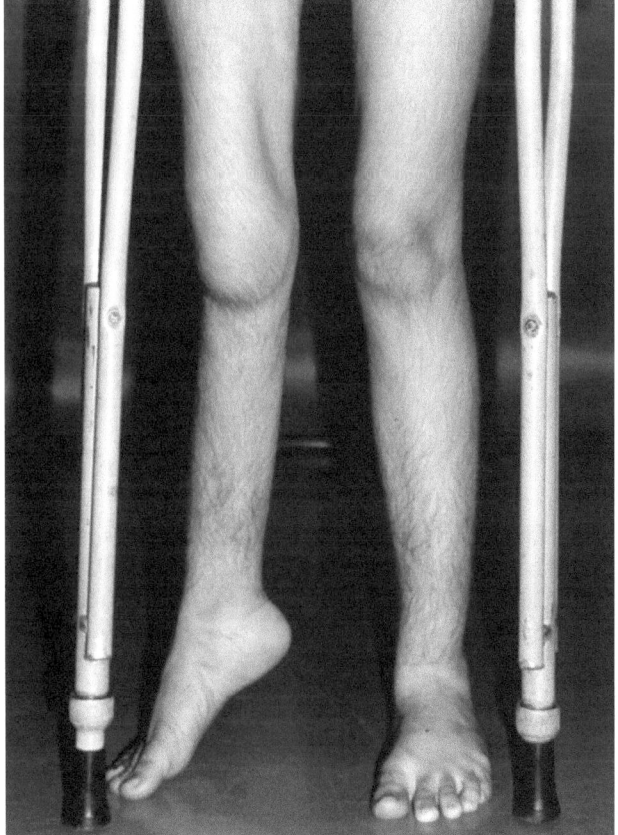

Fig. 5.2 External tibial torsion as a result of contracted ilio-tibial tract

medius and minimus, sartorius, rectus femoris, and the anterior hip capsule. Release must be followed by serial casting, with the hip in progressive adduction and extension and the knee straight.

Gluteal Paralysis

Weakness of hip abduction (gluteus medius and minimus) produces a positive Trendelenburg sign. This can be treated by the Mustard procedure [35]. When both gluteus medius and maximus are paralyzed, hip abduction and extension are weak. There is also forward tilting of the pelvis (backward body lurch) in addition to a Trendelenburg sign. Under such circumstances, the Sharrard transfer of ilio-psoas is preferred [36]. The ilio-psoas transfer forms part of the treatment of paralytic dislocation of hip in poliomyelitis. It should not be forgotten that hip flexion is weakened by the transfer.

Ilio-psoas transfer by the Mustard and Sharrard procedures is useful for patients with partial gluteal paralysis. It will improve stability during walking and thus the gait. Good abdominal muscle strength and a powerful sartorius, which becomes a primary hip flexor later, are important prerequisites.

The aim of the Mustard procedure is to transfer the ilio-psoas to augment hip abduction. The ilio-psoas, with its bony attachment, is isolated via a standard Smith–Peterson approach. The muscle is passed through a bony notch between the anterior superior and inferior iliac spines, to be attached to the greater trochanter. Post-operative immobilization of the hip in abduction is necessary.

In the Sharrard procedure, the ilio-psoas is transferred posterior and lateral to the hip joint through a large window in the ilium adjacent to the sacro-iliac joint [26, 27, 36]. The tendon is advanced through a tunnel in the greater trochanter to its anterolateral surface. This procedure is more extensive and technically more difficult than the Mustard procedure, but may be appropriate for patients with weakened hip extension. Prior anterior soft tissue release, abductor tenotomy and concomitant varus osteotomy of the hip may be required. From our experience, both transfers (Sharrard and Mustard) seldom produce strong abduction power but prevent the hip from redislocation by a tenodesis effect.

External Oblique Transfer

This muscle may be transferred to the greater trochanter in patients suffering from gluteus medius paralysis in whom the ilio-psoas is not suitable for transfer.

Tensor Fasciae Latae Transfer

This muscle can be transferred posteriorly for gluteus medius weakness and hip instability when no other muscles are suitable for transfer [27, 28].

Erector Spinae Transfer

This procedure is occasionally used for gluteus maximus weakness [37].

Paralytic Poliomyelitic Hip Subluxation and Dislocation

There are two groups of patients with subluxation or dislocation in poliomyelitis. The first group is due to muscle imbalance [38]. Initially, the hip adductors and flexors overpower the abductors and extensors. Subsequently, bony factors develop in the form of femoral neck valgus and increased anteversion. The acetabulum becomes shallow and oblique as the patient begins to bear weight, stretching the capsule, and allowing the femoral head to subluxate or dislocate. Pelvic obliquity aggravates this process, the hip on the higher side adducting and displacing (Fig. 5.3).

Both soft tissue and skeletal factors have to be dealt with. Concentric reduction of the hip is achieved by either closed or open reduction. Traction is often required for late cases before open reduction, especially after 3 years of age.

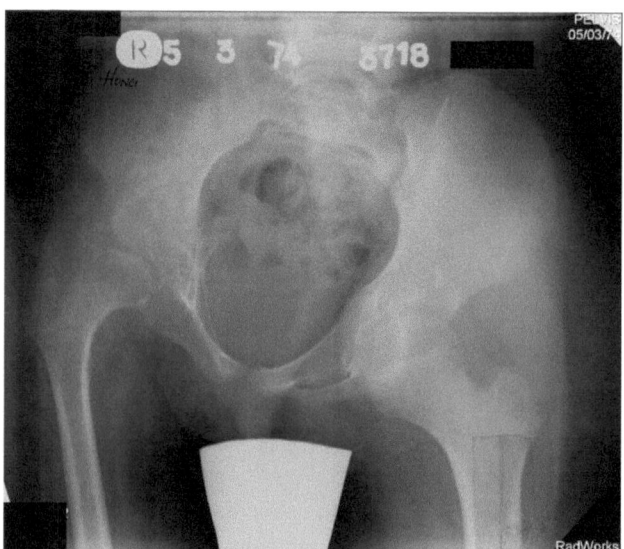

Fig. 5.3 Right hip subluxation. The right hip is adducted with resulting pelvic obliquity. Note the right hemipelvic and femoral hypoplasia

The muscle imbalance must be corrected by appropriate tendon transfers, but should be deferred until bony deformities have been corrected [38, 39]. Both upper femoral varus derotation osteotomy (sometimes with shortening of the femur to decrease the tension on the reduced femoral head) and acetabular reconstruction are required; alternatively, redirection by innominate osteotomy or increase in femoral head coverage by the use of a Chiari osteotomy may be indicated, depending upon the configuration of the acetabular defect. Acetabular reorientation procedures are often inappropriate because the acetabulum has "wandered" superiorly and laterally. Any associated predisposing cause of subluxation such as pelvic obliquity must be dealt with to prevent recurrence. Hip arthrodesis is seldom indicated for paralytic dislocation unless there is articular degeneration and painful impingement.

In the second group of patients, the hip subluxation or dislocation is provoked by pelvic obliquity with resulting poor coverage of the higher hip. Correcting the pelvic obliquity alone may improve the containment of the hip in some patients. Additional procedures to correct the excessive femoral anteversion and coxa valga and to improve the acetabular coverage may be needed if the reduction is still unsatisfactory after the pelvic obliquity is corrected.

The Flail Hip

Lack of muscle power around the hip is often associated with major paralysis distally. Multiple orthotic devices may be necessary to allow standing and walking. The flail hip seldom dislocates and is usually asymptomatic unless it is associated with pelvic obliquity, usually a sequel to paralytic lumbar scoliosis. Arthrodesis of a flail hip is associated with many disadvantages and is generally reserved as a salvage procedure. Sharp et al. [40] reported a high incidence of femoral fracture and pseudoarthrosis. Hallock showed good pain relief after hip fusion in poliomyelitic patients with arthritic hip subluxation or dislocation and improved stability in hips that have extensive muscle weakness [39, 41, 42].

Pelvic Obliquity

This can be produced by contracture above the pelvis when lumbar or thoraco-lumbar scoliosis is produced by asymmetrical paralysis of the quadratus lumborum and oblique abdominal muscles (Fig. 5.4). Below the pelvis, a contracture of the ilio-tibial tract causes ipsilateral downward tilting of the pelvis followed by contracture of the trunk muscles on the contralateral side. A lumbar scoliosis and hip subluxation are further aggravated by an adduction contracture with apparent shortening of the opposite leg. The

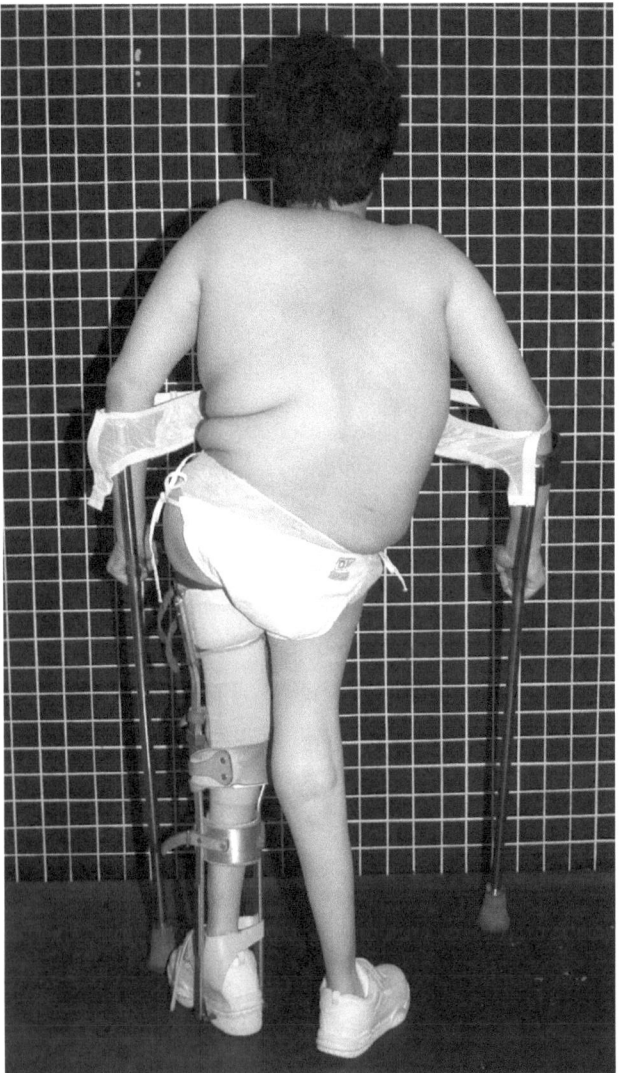

Fig. 5.4 This patient suffered from severe lumbar scoliosis with marked pelvic obliquity

treatment of pelvic obliquity is directed at the cause and any fixed secondary deformities, if present. [43] Lee, Choi, et al. [44] classified the pelvic obliquity in poliomyelitis into two major types and four subtypes depending upon the side of the shorter leg. In type I, the pelvis is lower on the side of the short leg and in type II it is raised. In type I, ipsilateral abductor release and contralateral lumbodorsal fasciotomy are recommended to correct the deformity. Type II deformities are less common. Contralateral abductor fasciotomy is undertaken first if an abduction contracture is present. This is followed by triple pelvic osteotomy with transiliac lengthening and ipsilateral lumbodorsal fasciotomy if the higher hip is not sufficiently stable or the correction of pelvic obliquity is inadequate.

The Knee

The most common deformity of the knee is fixed flexion deformity of varying severity. Other deformities are genu recurvatum, genu valgum, and, rarely, genu varum.

Knee Flexion Contracture

The causes of fixed flexion contracture include ilio-tibial tract contracture and quadriceps paralysis in the presence of normal hamstrings. Genu valgum and external rotation of the tibia coexist because of ilio-tibial tract contracture and a strong biceps femoris with weak medial hamstrings. Posterior subluxation of the tibia may also occur secondary to muscle imbalance. This is one of the factors limiting serial plaster correction of fixed-knee deformities so this technique should be used only in mild cases (Fig. 5.5) [45].

Knee flexion contracture places the knee at a mechanical disadvantage. The weak quadriceps fails to compensate for the loss of the locking mechanism that occurs in the slight knee hyperextension during the stance phase of gait. In order to prevent the knee buckling during walking, the patient may require a "hand on the knee" gait (Fig. 5.6). A Yount fasciotomy of the ilio-tibial tract may be necessary [34]. Flexion contracture of moderate to severe degree is difficult to treat. Secondary adaptive changes are present in the form of flattening of the articular surface and disproportionate increase in growth of the anterior portion of the tibia and femur compared with the posterior portion. This further increases the chance of posterior subluxation of the tibia upon the femur. Supracondylar osteotomy is preferred to soft tissue release in

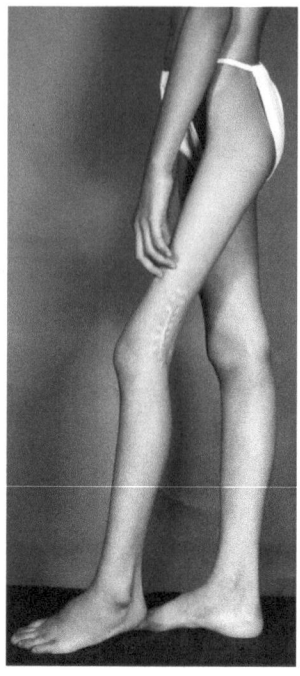

Fig. 5.6 Mild knee flexion contracture. The patient walked with a hand-on-knee gait

the presence of secondary bony changes; it can correct any valgus deformity that coexists [46].

Surgical correction of severe flexion contracture may require staged procedures; the results are usually better in children. Initial posterior capsulotomy and ilio-tibial tract release, including division of the posterior cruciate ligament, and skeletal traction or casting may be necessary. A supracondylar osteotomy with or without shortening of the bone is required in the second stage. A good range of knee flexion is important for success (Fig. 5.7) [46].

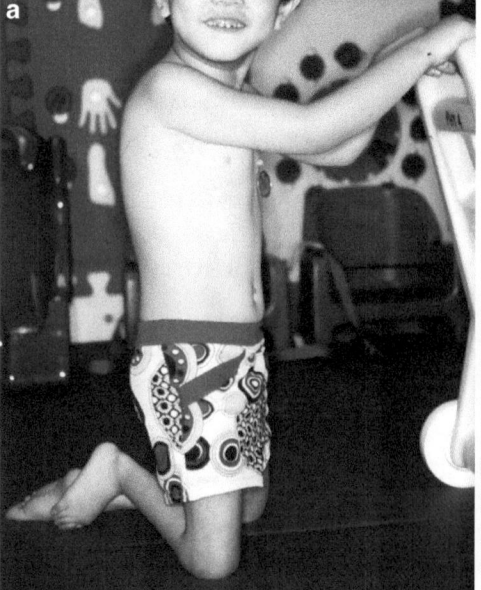
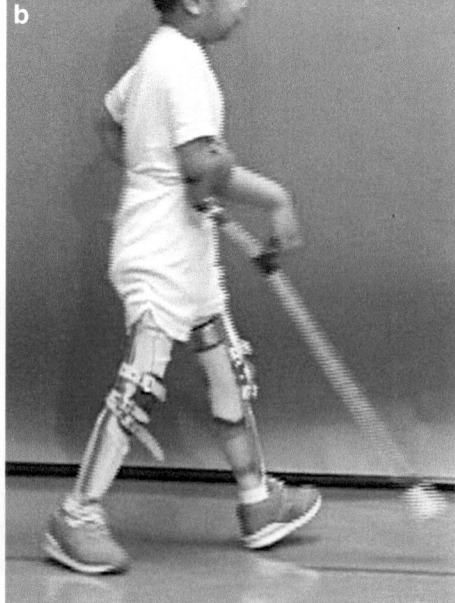

Fig. 5.5 (a) This boy had severe knee flexion contractures and had to walk on his knees. (b) He managed to walk with a pair of calipers after correction of the deformity

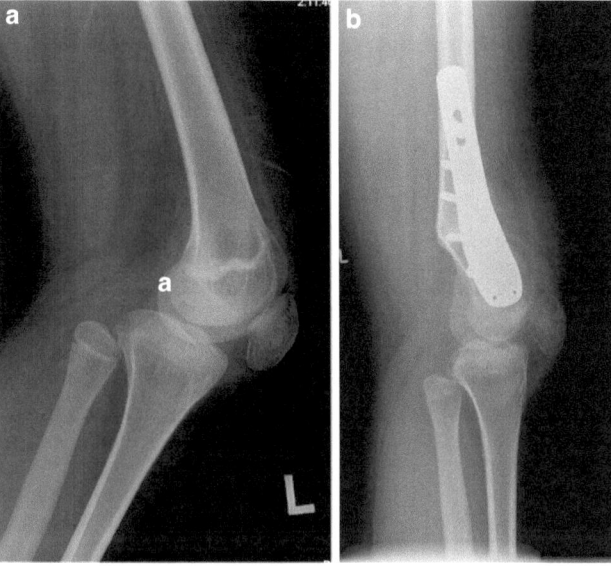

Fig. 5.7 (a) Knee flexion contracture was secondary to quadriceps weakness and was too severe to be corrected by soft tissue release alone. (b) Supracondylar extension osteotomy with plate and screws fixation to allow earlier mobilization. The knee is overcorrected to produce slight recurvatum which will improve the stability of the knee during stance

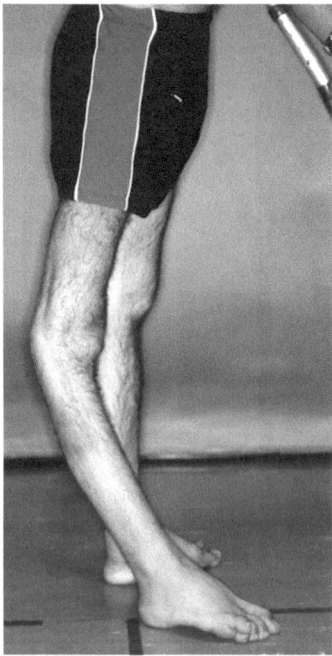

Fig. 5.8 Severe knee recurvatum

Genu Recurvatum

Mild genu recurvatum is common and is not disabling. In early cases, it results from overstretching of the posterior knee structures and later on, secondary bony changes occur with progressive flattening of the anterior aspect of both upper tibia and femoral condyles.

When the triceps surae is normal in the presence of paralysis of the quadriceps and hamstrings, the knee cannot be locked in neutral extension. The ground reaction force pushes the tibia posteriorly and the knee hyperextends in the stance phase of gait. The weight-bearing area of the knee joint is shifted anteriorly, and with time, the tibial plateau slopes downward and forward. This deformity can be corrected by wedge osteotomy of the proximal tibia. Mehta and Mukherjee [47] reported successful correction of the knee recurvatum with a distal femoral flexion osteotomy in patients with flattening of the anterior condyles.

When there is weakness in both the triceps surae and hamstrings, the knee hyperextends and the posterior structures stretch (Fig. 5.8). Gait is poor because of lack of push-off by the calf muscles. This type of recurvatum progresses more rapidly due to lack of dynamic support posteriorly, and early long-leg bracing is necessary [48]. Triple tenodesis, described by Perry et al. [49], utilizes the posterior capsule, semitendinosus, gracilis, biceps tendon, and the anterior half of ilio-tibial band and works well if the posterior soft tissues are protected until they are fully mature and any ankle equinus deformity corrected to the neutral position [49]. A

posterior tenodesis may stretch if used alone to block hyperextension of the knee. An anterior bone block utilizing the patella can be used to prevent progressive increase of hyperextension. Men et al. [50] reported long-term good results with the anterior bone block. Knee arthrodesis is usually considered as a salvage procedure.

Quadriceps paralysis is common. With adequate power of the hamstring and triceps surae or the presence of mild ankle equinus, the knee will be locked and stabilized in hyper extension in the stance phase of gait. Lengthening of the contracted triceps surae in a patient with quadriceps paralysis should be done cautiously as it may result in loss of this stabilization mechanism. Anterior hamstring transfer is reserved for the potentially brace-free patient with good hip flexion and extension power. The presence of an adequate triceps surae is essential to prevent the development of knee recurvatum deformity after the transfer. Transfer of both biceps femoris and semitendinosus is the preferred combination, although other muscles such as adductor longus and sartorius have also been utilized. Lateral dislocation of the patella is a troublesome complication following the transfer of biceps femoris alone [51, 52].

Flail Knee

The knee is very unstable and can be supported with an above-knee orthosis and a drop-lock. Arthrodesis will free the patient from the additional weight of an orthosis and is indicated for skeletally mature patients whose work is strenuous [53].

Foot and Ankle

A stable, plantigrade foot is required for normal walking. The foot affected by poliomyelitis may be unstable and muscle imbalance produces various combinations of deformity, which become structural with time. Plantar flexion/dorsiflexion imbalance produces equinus/calcaneus deformity at the ankle joint, whereas invertor/evertor imbalance produces varus/valgus deformity at the subtalar joint. Tendon release or transfer is useful and is the main method of treatment for a flexible deformity before bony maturity [27, 28, 54]. Bony resection and stabilization are indicated after skeletal maturity and are often best performed just before tendon transfer.

Dorsiflexor and Invertor Insufficiency

This is caused by tibialis anterior paralysis. The foot assumes an equinovalgus posture in the swing phase (Fig. 5.9). The proximal phalanges hyperextend and the metatarsal heads depress with resulting cock-up deformity due to overactivity of the toe extensors attempting to compensate for the loss of ankle dorsiflexion power. The unopposed triceps surae becomes contracted with resulting equinus deformity. The tibialis anterior dorsiflexes the first metatarsal and the peroneus longus plantar flexes it. Unopposed peroneus longus action will pronate the first ray and result in cavus deformity, the hindfoot being driven into varus during standing.

Early equinus can be corrected with intensive stretching of the tight structures behind the ankle followed by night time splintage. In more severe equinus deformity, posterior ankle capsulotomy and release of the subtalar joint are effective.

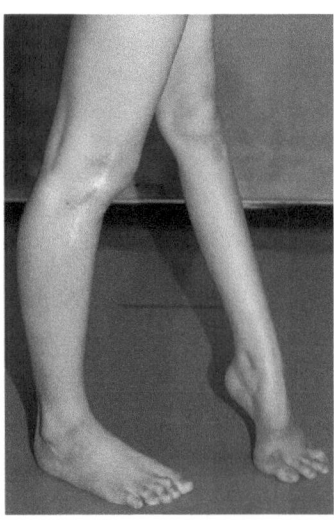

Fig. 5.9 Ankle equinus as a result of ankle dorsiflexor insufficiency

Lengthening of the Achilles tendon is best avoided whenever possible in order not to weaken the triceps surae. Loss of plantar flexion power results in major functional disability. Dorsiflexion power of the ankle can be restored with anterior transfer of the peroneus longus to the base of the second metatarsal. The peroneus brevis is sutured to the distal stump of peroneus longus to preserve its remaining tension on the first metatarsal. Active dorsiflexor power can be further improved by transferring the extensor digitorum longus to the dorsum of the midfoot or to the neck of the metatarsal for correction of claw toe deformity at the same time (Jones procedure).

Plantar release will improve the cavus deformity in early cases and first metatarsal or tarsal dorsal closing wedge osteotomy may be needed if secondary bony changes occur. If the deformity is associated with fixed hindfoot varus, it is corrected with a lateral closing wedge or lateral translation osteotomy of the os calcis. Joint fusion in the foot is avoided if possible to prevent the development of premature degeneration in adjacent joints. Good balancing of motor power across the joint by muscle transfer is important to achieve a good result and to prevent the recurrence of deformity. Triple arthrodesis (Lambrinudi modification) or subtalar joint fusion is needed if both peroneal tendons are utilized for transfer, thus avoiding subtalar instability.

Paralysis of tibialis anterior and tibialis posterior results in equinovalgus deformity. The peroneus longus is transferred to the base of the second metatarsal to replace the action of tibialis anterior. The flexor hallucis longus or flexor digitorum longus can be transferred to the tibialis posterior tendon.

Isolated tibialis posterior paralysis is rare. An eversion deformity results. Tendon transfer using flexor hallucis longus, flexor digitorum longus, or extensor hallucis longus has been successful.

Evertor Insufficiency

Isolated evertor insufficiency is rare. It usually occurs in association with paralysis of the long toe extensors and tibialis anterior.

In pure peroneal palsy, the hindfoot inverts and the forefoot adducts. The deforming force is the tibialis anterior which produces a dorsal elevation of the distal part of the first metatarsal and a dorsal bunion (Fig. 5.10). Lateral transfer of the tibialis anterior to the base of second metatarsal will correct a mild, flexible deformity. Fixed first metatarsal deformity requires osteotomy at its base, whereas hindfoot deformity requires a triple arthrodesis. Sometimes when the extensor hallucis longus overacts after tibialis anterior transfer, it may need transfer to the first metatarsal with interphalangeal fusion or tenodesis (Robert–Jones operation).

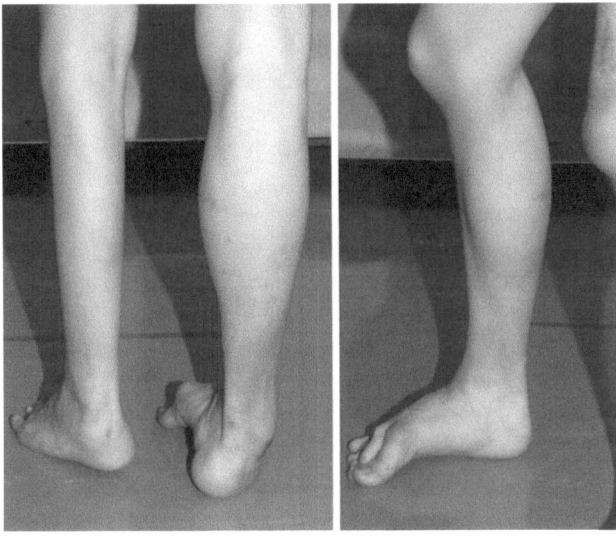

Fig. 5.10 Pes varus due to evertor insufficiency. The unopposed tibialis posterior inverts the hindfoot and the strong tibialis anterior elevates the first metatarsal and produces a dorsal bunion

Weakness of both peronei and long toe extensors produces a mild equinovarus deformity and treatment is the same as for pure evertor insufficiency. Paralysis of peronei, long toe extensors, and tibialis anterior produces a severe equinovarus deformity. The tibialis posterior and triceps surae are the deforming forces, and anterior transfer of the tibialis posterior to the base of the third metatarsal is effective. It may be augmented by prior soft tissue release of the cavus and anterior transfer of the long toe flexors.

Triceps Surae Paralysis

Triceps surae paralysis produces a calcaneus deformity. There is a lack of push-off during the gait cycle and the weight of the body cannot be transferred effectively to the metatarsal heads. Active ankle dorsiflexion, in the absence of a strong triceps surae, stretches the triceps surae and the posterior ankle capsule. The ankle joint is dorsiflexed with the head of talus and anterior part of os calcis displaced upward. The plantar flexors, namely, tibialis posterior, peronei, and long toe flexors, overact in an attempt to plantarflex the hindfoot, cause depression of the metatarsal heads, and produce a calcaneocavus deformity. The short toe flexors and plantar fascia will become contracted and act as a bowstring to pull the forefoot and os calcis together, resulting in further aggravation of the calcaneocavus deformity.

The posterior lever arm of the os calcis decreases as the os calcis become more dorsiflexed and vertical. This puts the weakened triceps surae in a mechanically unsounded position with further aggravation of dorsiflexion and plantar flexion imbalance. The loss of the normal contour of the heel results in a "pistol grip" deformity (Fig. 5.11).

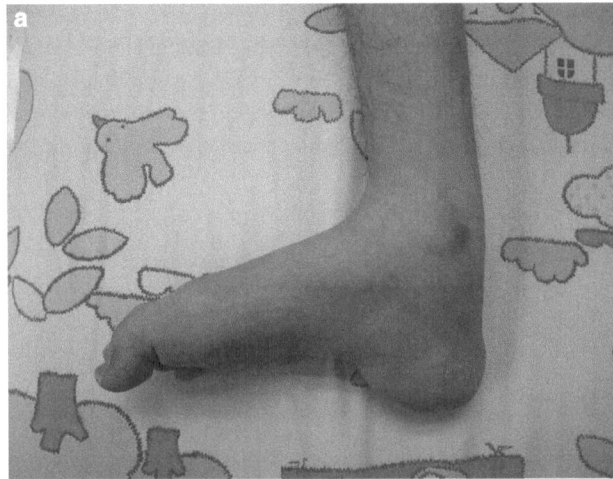
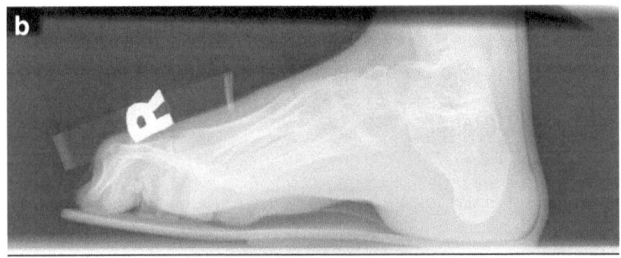

Fig. 5.11 (a) Calcaneal deformity with the typical "pistol grip" appearance due to weakness of triceps surae. (b) Radiograph of a calcaneal foot

Treatment of Calcaneus Ankle and Foot Deformities

Early splintage and a muscle exercise program are used to achieve maximal recovery of muscle power and to prevent the calcaneus deformity. An orthosis may be necessary to assist plantar flexion at the ankle and to limit dorsiflexion.

In the skeletally immature foot, "push-off" power can be helped by multiple tendon transfers such as tibialis posterior, the peronei and, rarely, tibialis anterior to the os calcis [55]. The plantar aponeurosis and intrinsic muscles should be released.

In the skeletally mature foot, bony resection and arthrodesis of the hindfoot are necessary before tendon transfer, usually after an interval of 6 weeks. With gross instability, a pantalar arthrodesis may be indicated. This is usually undertaken in patients with associated paralysis in order to eliminate the use of a caliper.

Tendon Transfer in Calcaneal Deformities

Invertor and evertor balance must be achieved during tendon transfer for calcaneal deformity. Calcaneocavus deformity is controlled by transfer of both peroneus brevis and tibialis posterior to the heel. Calcaneo-cavovalgus deformity requires transfer of both peronei. For the mobile calcaneal deformity, translocation of the peroneus longus into a groove on the posterior aspect of the os calcis is sometimes useful. The hamstrings have also been used to replace triceps surae function. Transfer of the tibialis anterior posteriorly through the interosseous membrane is advocated for younger patients with a flexible deformity [55].

Other Procedures for Calcaneal Foot Deformity

Calcaneal Osteotomy

Cavovarus deformity in a growing child may benefit from a calcaneal osteotomy. The os calcis can also be displaced posteriorly during the osteotomy [56].

Talectomy

This is indicated only when arthrodesis cannot be performed. The result is satisfactory for pain relief and cosmesis. Tibio-calcaneal fusion is necessary if talectomy fails [57, 58].

Elmslie's Procedure

This is a two-stage operation. Initially, soft tissue release and dorsal wedge excision of the talonavicular and calcaneocuboid joints correct the cavus deformity. This is followed by a second-stage posterior wedge excision of the subtalar joint, with the base of the wedge posteriorly to correct the calcaneal deformity. The Achilles tendon is shortened and tenodesed to the posterior aspect of the tibia. The long toe flexors are cut and sutured to the Achilles tendon.

Forefoot Equinus

A mobile forefoot equinus needs splintage only. Structural forefoot equinus deformity (plantaris) requires release of the plantar aponeurosis and wedge resection of the midfoot to enable the foot to be fitted with an orthosis.

Arthrodesis for Foot and Ankle Deformities

The most commonly practiced procedures are extra-articular subtalar arthrodesis and triple arthrodesis. Bone block procedures and ankle arthrodesis are now seldom performed.

Extra-articular Subtalar Arthrodesis

The Grice–Green extra-articular subtalar arthrodesis aims to correct hindfoot valgus in the supple foot (Fig. 5.12) [6, 59, 60]. The procedure was performed in young children to preserve the growth potential of the foot by avoiding injury to the preosseous cartilage. A tibial cortical graft was used as the strut in the sinus tarsi with good initial results. Graft complications and unsatisfactory later results led to the introduction of modifications of the original procedure with improved fixation and graft sources. A fibular graft inserted from the neck of talus through the sinus tarsi was devised by Batchelor, but a high rate of nonunion has been reported (Fig. 5.13) [61–65]. Dennyson and Fulford modified the Batchelor procedure by replacing the fibular graft with a screw and adding cancellous grafts into the sinus tarsi [66]. A combined Batchelor–Grice technique, using cancellous graft from the iliac crest with a fibular graft, was reported by Jaffray et al. [67] to achieve a 96% union rate and eliminated problems related to the presence of a screw (Fig. 5.14). The modified procedures reduced the occurrence of post-operative hindfoot varus deformity, which can produce a painful callosity over the lateral border of the foot.

Mosca has popularized the calcaneal lengthening osteotomy (first described by Evans in 1975) as an alternative for treatment of hindfoot valgus in neuromuscular patients [68]. However, in the authors' unpublished series of similar procedures, some loss of early correction was seen at mid-term follow-up. The procedure preserves the mobility of the subtalar joints and theoretically should reduce the

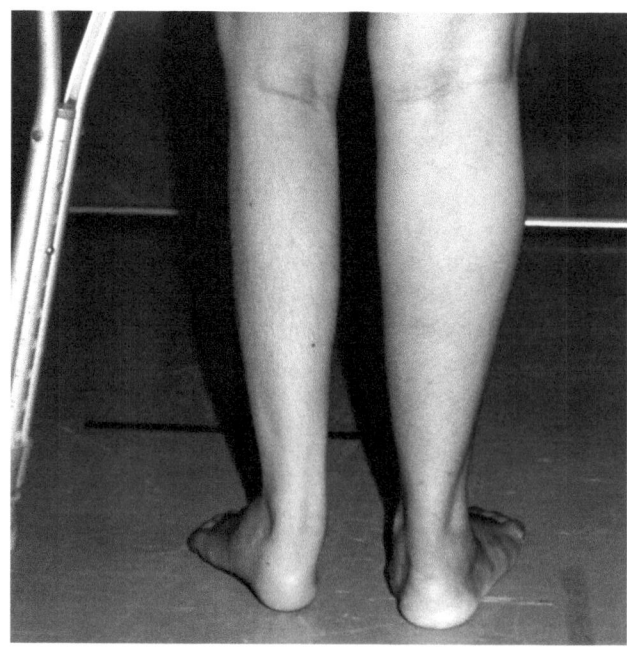

Fig. 5.12 Planovalgus deformity due to weakness of tibialis posterior

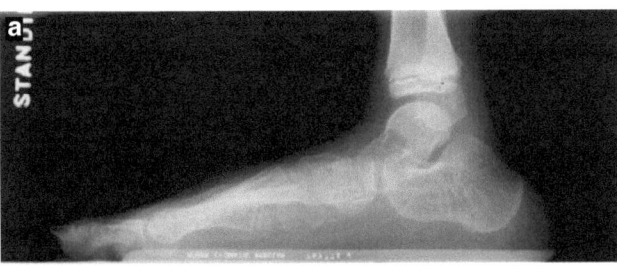

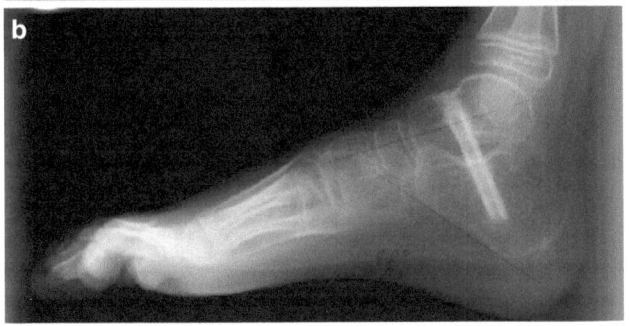

Fig. 5.13 (**a**) Radiographs of planovalgus foot. Note the increase of the talocalcaneal angle. (**b**) Batchelor type of extra-articular subtalar fusion. The fibular graft is inserted through the neck of talus

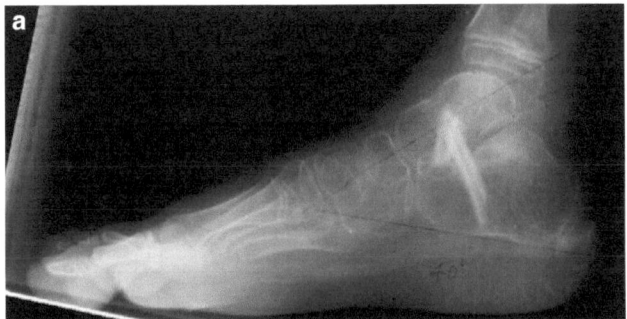

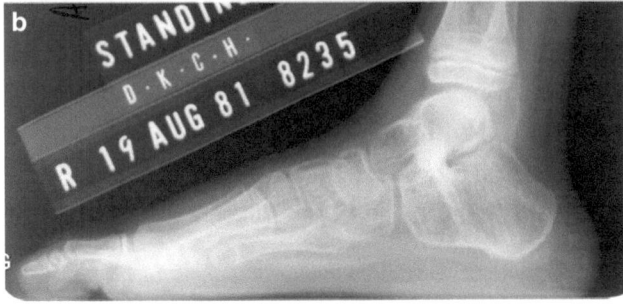

Fig. 5.14 (**a**) Combined Batchelor–Grice extra-articular subtalar fusion. Cortico-cancellous graft is inserted into the sinus tarsi in addition to the fibular graft. (**b**) Radiograph at 1 year after surgery. Note the fusion mass at sinus tarsi

incidence of adjacent joint degeneration. The procedure is not suitable in patients with complete paralysis or significant imbalance of the ankle invertors and evertors which cannot be corrected.

Standing radiographs of the foot and ankle are necessary to determine the site of the valgus deformity, which is occasionally present in the ankle.

Triple Arthrodesis

This operation is frequently performed for equinovalgus or varus deformity after the child has reached the age of 10 years [69]. The subtalar, calcaneocuboid, and talonavicular joints are resected and arthrodesed. Bony wedges are taken out to produce a plantigrade foot. Modifications of this procedure include posterior displacement of the foot to improve the mechanical advantage of the weakened triceps surae and the Lambrinudi arthrodesis for severe and rigid equinus deformity [70]. Any rotational malalignment of the limb must be considered before the triple arthrodesis in order to avoid malalignment of the foot during the procedure. The talonavicular joint is prone to nonunion and avascular necrosis of the talus may occur because of excessive resection [69]. The pseudoarthrosis rate has been reduced significantly in later reports because of improved fixation techniques. Residual deformity is not uncommon but does not result in significant symptoms. Late osteoarthritis of the ankle and midtarsal joints may develop secondary to stiffening of the hindfoot and ankle ligament laxity [71]. Although recurrence of hindfoot deformity is rare, secondary forefoot deformity may occur because of muscle imbalance. Nowadays, multiple osteotomies to correct the midfoot and hindfoot deformities are preferred to triple arthrodesis. The procedure is reserved for salvage in recurrent deformities and in chronic foot deformities associated with degenerative changes. For recurrent and severe deformities, gradual correction following osteotomies with the Ilizarov external fixation has been advocated [72].

Ankle and Pantalar Arthrodesis

Both procedures are seldom performed for poliomyelitis [69]. The flail foot is an indication for such a fusion and it will eliminate the need for an orthosis. A strong gluteus maximus (to extend the hip) and good hamstrings and posterior knee capsule (to prevent hyperextension of the knee) are prerequisites. The ankle has to be fused in 5° of equinus which will help to keep the knee in slight hyperextension during stance. A preoperative weight-bearing lateral radiograph will demonstrate talar subluxation in cases where pantalar arthrodesis is indicated.

Toes

There are three common causes for claw toe deformity (hyperextension of the metatarsophalangeal joint and flexion of the interphalangeal joints):

1. Loss of ankle dorsiflexion. The clawing is noticeable during the swing phase, as the long toe extensors try to compensate for the loss of ankle dorsiflexion power. Restoration of ankle dorsiflexion cures the clawing if it is still mobile.
2. Loss of ankle plantar flexion. The clawing is noticeable during stance phase, as the long toe flexors try to compensate for loss of ankle plantar flexion power. Restoration of active plantar flexion will eliminate the clawing.
3. Clawing associated with a cavus foot. The prime object is to treat the cavus. Intrinsic weakness is often present.

Clawing of the big toe can be dealt with by transferring the extensor hallucis longus tendon to the neck of the first ray (Jones operation). The interphalangeal joint of the big toe needs to be arthrodesed [73].

Clawing of the other toes as a result of the long toe flexors overacting may need a flexor to extensor transfer.

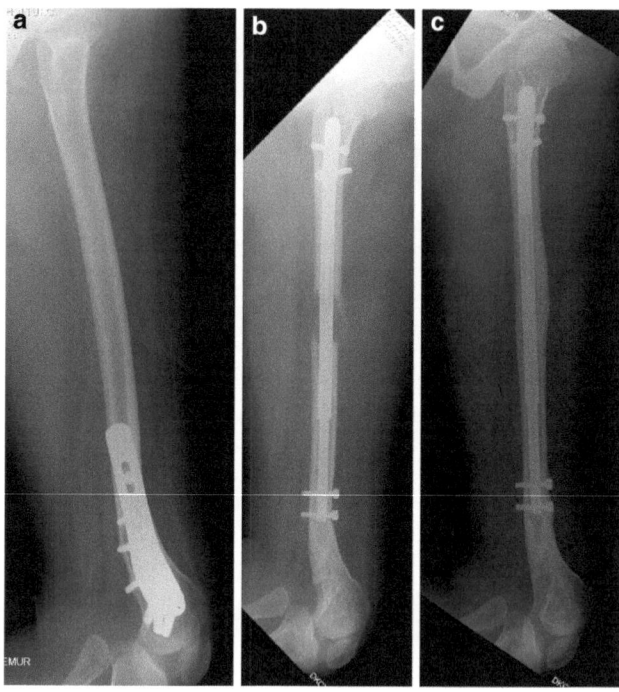

Fig. 5.15 (**a**) This patient had a previous supracondylar osteotomy for knee flexion contracture. She has 4.5 cm of left lower limb shortening (**b**) Femoral lengthening of 4 cm with intramedullary skeletal kinetic device in process. (**c**) Radiograph 1 year after surgery

Leg Length Discrepancy

Leg length discrepancy is common in patients with poliomyelitis [74, 75]. The limb shortening can be apparent due to pelvic obliquity and deformity of the limb. The treatment of apparent leg length discrepancy should be directed to the deformity and its correction should be carefully planned, taking into consideration the effects of the deformity upon gait. True leg length discrepancy is usually the result of asymmetric involvement of the lower limbs. From the authors' experience, leg lengthening in selected patients will improve the gait (Fig. 5.15). It is important to remember that the ankle equinus which originally compensated for the shortening should not be corrected past neutral if the quadriceps muscle is weak.

Post-poliomyelitis Syndrome

The post-poliomyelitis syndrome is characterized by the development of new muscle weakness, muscle fatigability, pain, and depression in patients who have recovered from paralytic poliomyelitis. The patients should have suffered from poliomyelitis with partial or complete neurological recovery but recovered sufficiently to enjoy good function and neurological stability for several decades (usually more

than 20 years) [76]. The diagnosis is made after other medical, orthopaedic, and neurological conditions are excluded. The prevalence reported in the literature is 20–80%.

The exact pathogenesis of the syndrome is still not certain [77–80]. The most likely cause is distal degeneration of the enlarged post-poliomyelitis motor unit. Ageing, with motor neuron loss, overuse, and disuse could be the contributing factors. Viral replication and reactivation have been suggested but have never been confirmed.

There is no specific treatment for the syndrome. Drugs such as pyridostigmine and steroids have been tried in randomized studies with no proven effect on the improvement of the symptoms. A multidisciplinary approach with emphasis upon muscle strengthening, the use of assistive devices in daily activities, and control of body weight may help to manage the symptoms. Intermittent breaks can be introduced into daily activities. Physical training has been recommended to counteract fatigue but may itself worsen the weakness.

Spinal Deformity

Scoliosis is a common sequel of poliomyelitis [81, 82]. Kyphosis is relatively rare. Post-poliomyelitic scoliosis is due to imbalance between the trunk and the intercostal muscles in the growing child. Curvature can be due to asymmetrical paralysis of trunk muscles or extensive symmetrical paralysis resulting in a collapsing spine. Six types of curves are commonly seen:

1. High thoracic curve: this is extremely unsightly and the prognosis is poor.
2. Thoracic curve: this is usually a long curve associated with an angular rib hump.
3. Lumbar curve: this is usually associated with pelvic obliquity, impaired sitting balance, and asymmetric ischial pressure. The hip on the high side may subluxate.
4. Double major curve: this is uncommon.
5. Long C curve: the entire trunk is involved, with the apex at the thoraco-lumbar junction.
6. Collapsing spine: the entire trunk sags because of extensive muscle involvement and the effect of gravity. The patient supports himself on the upper limbs holding onto the bed. Pelvic obliquity may be present.

Indications for Surgical Treatment

Most moderate to severe curves require surgery. Bracing is poorly tolerated and acts as a passive holding device only. Patients with profound weakness of the lower limb manage to walk with trick movement of the trunk. Patients have to be alerted to the possibility that the walking ability may deteriorate after the spine is fused. Before surgery, the following should be considered.

Age

The ideal time for surgery is just before the adolescent growth spurt, when most progression is expected. An extensive fusion is usually necessary because of the nature of the curve.

Curve Pattern

High thoracic curves need early fusion. The collapsing spine tends to remain flexible but should be fused when flexibility decreases or if upper limb function is grossly impaired and is no longer able to support the trunk. A mild thoracic, thoraco-lumbar, lumbar, or double major curve should be treated according to the same principles as idiopathic curves.

Progression

Curves of more than 40–50° that progress despite adequate bracing require surgical correction and fusion.

Pelvic Obliquity

Obliquity of more than 30° disturbs sitting balance and causes hip dislocation and asymmetrical ischial pressure. Surgical correction and fusion are indicated.

Method of Treatment

Preoperative casting has largely been abandoned because it is uncomfortable and causes further pulmonary impairment. The results of spinal surgery in poliomyelitis without internal fixation showed considerable loss of correction at final follow-up and a high pseudoarthrosis rate. Multiple operations were usually required. By contrast, the use of internal fixation has markedly improved correction and maintenance of correction at long-term follow-up. The most popular posterior instrumentation 30 years ago was the Harrington system, with or without sublaminar wiring, followed by 3–6 months of casting until radiological fusion was achieved. This was associated with high rate of pseudoarthrosis so that subsequently techniques of combined anterior and posterior instrumentation were developed with significant improvement in fusion rates [81–86]. Nowadays, segmental instrumentation with wires, hooks, and screws has become the standard procedure for paralytic scoliosis, giving a more stable fixation. This allows better correction of the curve with increased fusion rates; post-operative bracing is usually unnecessary. Combined anterior and posterior instrumentation is used in severe and rigid curves, especially with severe pelvic obliquity [44, 81, 82, 84, 87].

Preoperative halo-pelvic/halo-femoral traction can be useful in the treatment of the poliomyelitic spine undergoing corrective surgery, especially when staged anterior and posterior surgery are contemplated. This combined method is useful for long lumbar C curves, collapsing spines, and severe long thoracic curves (89). Combined anterior and posterior fusion down to the sacrum reduces the chance of pseudoarthrosis. Anterior instrumentation down to L5 provides maximum correction of pelvic obliquity. Curves above 100° or between 80° and 100° with rigidity will benefit from preoperative halo-pelvic traction. Long C curves, collapsing spines, and lumbar curves with pelvic obliquity should always be fused to the sacrum.

References

1. Anonymous. Poliomyelitis in 1977, Notes and News. WHO Chron 1979; 33:63–70.
2. World Health Organization. Poliomyelitis. Fact sheet #114. At: http://www.who.int/mediacentre/factsheets/fs114/en/index.html. Accessed 19 Sep. 2008.

3. Strebel PM, Sutter RW, Cochi SL, et al. Epidemiology of poliomyelitis in the United States one decade after the last reported case of indigenous wild virus-associated disease. Clin Infect Dis 1992; 14:568.

4. Sabin AB. Oral poliovirus vaccine. History of its development and prospects. Eradication of poliomyelitis. JAMA 1965; 194:872–881.

5. Diveley RL. Anterior poliomyelitis: A study of the acute stage with special reference to the early diagnosis and treatment. J Bone Joint Surg Am 1929; 11:100–122.

6. Green WT, Grice DS. The management of chronic poliomyelitis. AAOS Instr Course Lect 1952; 9:85–90.

7. Lenhard RE. Prognosis in poliomyelitis. J Bone Joint Surg Am 1950; 32:71–79.

8. Mayer L. The physiologic method of tendon transplants. Reviewed after forty years. AAOS Instr Course Lect 1956; 13: 116–121.

9. Kumar K, Kapahtia NK. The pattern of muscle involvement in poliomyelitis of the upper limb. Int Orthop 1986; 10:11–15.

10. Bennett JB, Allan CH. Tendon transfers about the shoulder and elbow in obstetrical brachial plexus palsy. J Bone Joint Surg 1999; 81-A:1612–1627.

11. Kotwal PP, Mittal R, Malhotra R. Trapezius transfer for deltoid paralysis. J Bone Joint Surgery Br 1998; 80-B:114–116.

12. Saha AK. Surgery of the paralysed and flail shoulder. Acta Orthop Scand Supplement 1967; 97:7–90 .

13. Saha AK. Surgical rehabilitation of paralyzed shoulder following poliomyelitis in adults and children. J Int Coll Surg 1964; 42:198.

14. Brockway A. An operation to improve abduction power of the shoulder in poliomyelitis. J Bone Joint Surg Am 1939; 21:451–455.

15. Harmon PH. Anterior transplantation of the posterior deltoid for shoulder palsy and dislocation in poliomyelitis. Surg Gynecol Obstet 1947; 84:117.

16. American Orthopaedic Association—Research Committee: A survey of end results on stabilization of the paralytic shoulder. J Bone and Joint Surg 1942; 24:699–707.

17. May VR Jr. Shoulder Fusion. A Review of Fourteen Cases. J. Bone and Joint Surg 1962; 44-A:65–76.

18. De Velasco Polo G, Monterrubio AC. Arthrodesis of the Shoulder. Clin Orthop 1973; 90:178–182.

19. Mah JY, Hall JE. Arthrodesis of the shoulder in children. J Bone Joint Surg Am 1990; 72:582–586.

20. Rowe CR. Re-evaluation of the Position of the Arm in Arthrodesis of the Shoulder in the Adult. J Bone and Joint Surg Am 1974; 56:913–922.

21. Steindler A. Muscle and tendon transplant at the elbow. AAOS Instr Course Lect Reconstr Surg 1944; 2:276–282.

22. Carroll RE, Hill NA. Triceps transfer to restore elbow flexion. J Bone Joint Surg Am 1970; 52:239.

23. Clark JMP. Reconstruction of biceps brachii by pectoral muscle transplantation. Br J Surg 1946; 34:180.

24. Irwin CE, Eyler DL. Surgical rehabilitation of the hand and forearm disabled by poliomyelitis. J Bone Joint Surg Am 1951; 33:825–835.

25. Schnute WJ, Tachdjian MO. Intermetacarpal bone block for thenar paralysis following poliomyelitis: An end-result study. J Bone Joint Surg Am 1963; 45:1663–1670.

26. Sharrard WJW. Distribution of permanent paralysis of lower limbs in poliomyelitis—a clinical and pathological study. J Bone Joint Surg 1955; 37 B:540.

27. Sharrard WJW. Paediatric Orthopaedics and Fractures. 2nd ed. Oxford, London: Blackwell Scientific; 1979:889.

28. Watts HG. Orthopedic techniques in the management of the residua of paralytic poliomyelitis. Techn Orthop 2005; 20(2):179–189.

29. Ober FR. The role of iliotibial band and fascia lata as a factor in the causation of low-back disabilities and sciatica. J Bone Joint Surg Am 1936; 18:105–110.

30. Green NE, Griffin PP. Hip dysplasia associated with abduction contracture of the contralateral hip J Bone Joint Surg Am 1982; 64:1273–1281.

31. Asirvatham R, Watts HG, Rooney RJ. Rotation osteotomy of the tibia after poliomyelitis. J Bone Joint Surgery Br 1990; 72-B:409–11.

32. Irwin CE. The iliotibial band: Its role in producing deformity in poliomyelitis. J Bone Joint Surg Am 1949; 31:141.

33. McNicol D, Leong JCY, Hsu LCS. Supramalleolar Derotation Osteotomy for Lateral tibial torsion and associated equino-varus deformity of the foot. J Bone Joint Surg Br 1983; 65: 166–170.

34. Yount CC. The role of the tensor fasciae femoris in certain deformities of the lower extremities. J Bone Joint Surg. 1926; 8:171–177.

35. Mustard WT. A follow-up study of iliopsoas transfer for hip instability. J Bone Joint Surg 1959; 41B:289–293.

36. Sharrard WJW. Posterior iliopsoas transplantation in the treatment of paralytic dislocation of the hip. J Bone Joint Surg 1964; 46B:426–434.

37. Hogshead HP, Ponseti IV. Fascia lata transfer to the erector spinae for the treatment of flexion-abduction contractures of the hip in patients with poliomyelitis and meningomyelocele: Evaluation of results. J Bone Joint Surg Am 1964; 46:1389.

38. Lau JHK, Parker JC, Hsu LCS, Leong JCY. Paralytic hip instability in poliomyelitis. J Bone Joint Surg 1986; 68B:528–533.

39. Hallock H. Surgical stabilization of dislocated paralytic hips: End-results study. Surg Gynecol Obstet 1942; 75:742.

40. Sharp NN, Guhl JF, Sorensen RI, et al. Hip fusion in poliomyelitis in children: A preliminary report. J Bone Joint Surg Am 1964; 46:121–133.

41. Hallock H. Arthrodesis of the hip for instability and pain in poliomyelitis. J Bone Joint Surg Am 1950; 2:904.

42. Hallock H. Hip arthrodesis in poliomyelitis. Bull N Y Hosp 1958; 2:18.

43. O'Brien JP, Dwyer AP, Hodgson AR. A paralytic pelvic obliquity. J Bone Joint Surg 1975; 57A:626–632.

44. Lee DY, Choi IH, Chung CY, et al. Fixed pelvic obliquity after poliomyelitis. J Bone Joint Surg 1997; 79:190.

45. Hughes RE, Risser JC. The correction of knee-flexion deformity, after poliomyelitis, by wedging plasters. J Bone Joint Surg Am 1934; 16:935–946.

46. Leong JCY, Alade CO, Fang D. Supracondylar femoral osteotomy for knee flexion contracture resulting from poliomyelitis. J Bone Joint Surgery 1982; 64-B:198–201.

47. Mehta SN, Mukherjee AK. Flexion osteotomy of the femur for genu recurvatum after poliomyelitis. J Bone Joint Surg Br 1991; 73:200.

48. Heyman CH. Operative treatment of paralytic genu recurvatum. J Bone Joint Surg Am 1962; 44:1246.

49. Perry J, O'Brien JP, Hodgson AR. Triple tenodesis of the knee: a soft-tissue operation for the correction of paralytic genu recurvatum. J Bone Joint Surg 1976; 58-A:978–985.

50. Men HX, Bian CH, Yang CD, et al. Surgical treatment of the flail knee after poliomyelitis. J Bone Joint Surg Br 1991; 73-B:195–199.

51. Broderick TF, Reidy JA, Barr JS. Tendon transplantations in the lower extremity: A review of end results in poliomyelitis II. Tendon transplantations at the knee. J Bone Joint Surg Am 1952; 34:909–914.

52. Crego Jr CH, Fischer FJ. Transplantation of the biceps femoris for the relief of quadriceps femoris paralysis in residual poliomyelitis. J Bone Joint Surg 1931; 13:515.

53. Cleveland M. Operative fusion of the unstable or flail knee due to anterior poliomyelitis: A study of the late results. J Bone Joint Surg Am 1932; 14:525–534.

54. Emmel HE, Le Cocq JF. Hamstring transplant for the prevention of calcaneocavus foot in poliomyelitis. J Bone Joint Surg Am 1958; 40:911–917.

55. Hsu LCS, Swanson L, Leong JCY, Low WD. Telemetric electromyographic analysis of muscles transferred to the os calcis in paralysed limbs. Clin Orthop 1985; 201:71–74.

56. Pandey AK, Pandey S, Prasad V. Calcaneal osteotomy and tendon sling for the management of calcaneus deformity. J Bone Joint Surg Am 1989; 71:1192–1198.

57. Legaspi J, Li YH, Chow W, Leong JCY. Talectomy in patients with recurrent deformity in club foot. A long-term follow-up study. J Bone Joint Surg 2001; 83B:384–387.

58. Nicomedez FPI, Li YH, Leong JCY. Tibiocalcaneal fusion after talectomy in arthrogrypotic patients. J Pediatr Orthoped 2003; 23(5):654–657.

59. Grice DS. An extra-articular arthrodesis of the subastragalar joint for correction of paralytic flat feet in children. J Bone Joint Surg Am 1952; 34-A:927–940.

60. Seymour N, Evans DK. A modification of the Grice subtalar arthrodesis. J Bone Joint Surg Br 1968; 50-B:372–375.

61. Hsu LCS, O'Brien JP, Yau ACMC, Hodgson AR. Batchelor's extra-articular subtalar arthrodesis: A report on sixty-four procedures in patients with poliomyelitic deformities. J Bone Joint Surg Am 1976; 58-A:243–247.

62. Hsu LCS, O'Brien JP, Yau ACMC, Hodgson AR. Valgus deformity of the ankle in children with fibular pseudarthrosis. J Bone Joint Surg Am 1974; 56-A:503–510.

63. Bhan S, Malhotra R. Subtalar arthrodesis for flexion hindfoot deformities in children. Arch Orthop Trauma Surg 1998; 117:312–315.

64. Brown A. A simple method of fusion of the subtalar joint in children. J Bone Joint Surg Br 1968; 50-B:369–371.

65. Hsu LCS, Yau ACMC, O'Brien JP, Hodgson AR. Valgus deformity of the ankle resulting from fibular resection for a graft in subtalar fusion in children. J Bone Joint Surg Am 1972; 54-A:585–594.

66. Dennyson WG, Fulford GE. Subtalar arthrodesis by cancellous grafts and metallic internal fixation. J Bone Joint Surg Br 1976; 58-B:507–510.

67. Jaffray D, Hsu L, Leong JCY. The Batchelor-Grice extra-articular subtalar arthrodesis. J Bone Joint Surg 1986; 68-B:125–127.

68. Mosca VS. Calcaneal lengthening for valgus deformity of the hindfoot. Results in children who had severe, symptomatic flatfoot and skewfoot. J Bone Joint Surg Am 1995; 77:500–512.

69. Crego CH, McCarroll HR. Recurrent deformities in stabilized paralytic feet: A report of 1100 consecutive stabilizations in poliomyelitis. J Bone Joint Surg Am 1938; 20:609–620.

70. Tang SC, Leong JCY, Hsu LCS. Lambrinudi triple arthrodesis for correction of severe rigid drop-foot. J Bone Joint Surg 1984; 66B:66–72.

71. Saltzman CL, Fehrle MJ, Cooper RR, et al. Triple arthrodesis: Twenty-five and forty-four-year average follow-up of the same patients. J Bone Joint Surg 1999; 81-A:1391–1402.

72. Kong KFJ, Li YH, Kwok HY. Treatment of foot deformities in children by Ilizarov method. Proceedings, the 19th Annual Congress of the Hong Kong Orthopaedic Association. 1999: 61

73. Jones R. The soldier's foot and the treatment of common deformities of the foot. Part III Claw foot. Br Med J 1916; I:749.

74. Aldegheri R. Distraction osteogenesis for lengthening of the tibia in patients who have limb-length discrepancy or short stature. J Bone Joint Surg Am 1999; 81:624–634.

75. Macnicol MF, Catto AM. Twenty-year review of tibial lengthening for poliomyelitis. J Bone Joint Surg 1982; 64B:607–610.

76. Perry J, Fontaine JD, Mulroy S. Findings in post-poliomyelitis syndrome. Weakness of muscles of the calf as a source of late pain and fatigue of muscles of the thigh after poliomyelitis. J Bone Joint Surg Am 1995; 77:1148–1153.

77. Farbu E. Post-polio syndrome—diagnosis and management. ACNR 2005; 5:10–11.

78. Lin KH, Lim YW. Post-poliomyelitis syndrome: Case report and review of the literature. Ann Acad Med Singapore 2005; 34:447–449.

79. Nollet F. Post-polio syndrome. Orphanet Encyclopedia; 2004:2–8. At http://www.orpha.net/data/patho/GB/uk-PP.pdf. Accessed 02 October 2008.

80. Trojan DA, Cashman NR. Post-poliomyelitis syndrome. Muscle Nerve 2005; 31:6–19.

81. Leong JCY, Wilding K, Mok CK, et al. Surgical treatment of scoliosis following poliomyelitis. J Bone Joint Surg 1981; 3A:726–732.

82. Leong JCY, Hsu LCS. Poliomyelitis of the spine. In: McCollister Evarts C, ed. Surgery of the Musculoskeletal System, 2nd ed. New York: Churchill Livingstone; 1990:2049–2072.

83. Eberle CF. Failure of fixation after segmental spinal instrumentation without arthrodesis in the management of paralytic scoliosis. J Bone Joint Surg Am 1988; 70:696.

84. Hsu LCS, Cheng CL, Leong JCY. Treatment of severe poliomyelitis spinal deformity after failed posterior fusion. J West Paci Orthop Assoc 1985; 22(2):27–33.

85. Mayer PJ, Dove J, Ditmanson M, et al. Post-poliomyelitis paralytic scoliosis. A review of curve patterns and results of surgical treatments in 118 consecutive patients. Spine 1981; 6:573.

86. Pavon SJ, Manning C. Posterior spinal fusion for scoliosis due to anterior poliomyelitis. J Bone Joint Surg 1970; 52-B:420–431.

87. O'Brien JP, Yau AC, Gertzbein S, Hodgson AR. Combined staged anterior and posterior correction and fusion of the spine in scoliosis following poliomyelitis. Clin Orthop Rel Res 1975b; 110:81–111.

Chapter 6

Orthopaedic Management of Cerebral Palsy

James E. Robb and Reinald Brunner

Definition

Ingram has provided a suitable description:

> Cerebral palsy is used as an inclusive term to describe a group of non-progressive disorders occurring in young children in which disease of the brain causes impairment of motor function. Impairment of motor function may be the result of paresis, involuntary movement, or incoordination, but motor dysfunctions which are transient, or are the result of progressive disease of the brain, or attributable to abnormalities of the spinal cord, are excluded. [1].

All children with cerebral palsy (CP) are "brain-damaged" and have associated disabilities such as epilepsy (33%), mental handicap (19–50%), speech disorders (25–80%), behavioral disturbances, specific learning difficulties, or abnormal visual perception (34–58%) [2]. The likelihood of significant visual deficits is greater in children with higher gross motor function classification system (GMFCS) scores, independent of gestational age [3]. Sensory deficits are also present and Sanger and Kukke have shown that children with secondary dystonia and diplegia due to CP have deficits of tactile sensation [4]. An appropriate sensory input is a prerequisite for an adequate motor control. While the neurological damage may be non-progressive, CP is certainly a progressive orthopaedic condition, which may be influenced by growth or intervention. The condition is rarely manifest at birth but presents later as developmental delay.

Classification

This may be

1. Topographical: hemiplegia, diplegia, and total body involvement (tetraplegia).
2. Neurological: spastic, athetoid, ataxic, rigid, or mixed.

J.E. Robb (✉)
Department of Orthopaedic Surgery, Royal Hospital for Sick Children, Edinburgh, UK; University of Edinburgh, Edinburgh, UK; University of St. Andrews, Edinburgh, UK

Classification based on severity is difficult because of the inaccuracy of quantifying the severity of spasticity, athetosis, or ataxia. Some children fit into typical patterns, but others do not and often there is an overlap. The term "total body involvement" is preferred to tetraplegia as it embraces the concept of impaired head and trunk control.

Incidence

Cerebral palsy occurs in approximately 0.25% of all live births and in the majority no cause can be identified. It was commonly thought that the disorder resulted from brain asphyxia due to problems during labor, but despite advances in obstetric care, the incidence has remained constant in the recent past. However, the pattern of CP has changed in that there has been a notable decrease in athetosis due to erythroblastosis fetalis. In a multicenter study which involved approximately 54,000 births, Nelson and Ellenberg found that only 21% of the 189 children who developed CP had any sign of intra-partum asphyxia and 9% had evidence of asphyxia in the absence of congenital malformation [5]. Maternal mental retardation, a birthweight below 2 kg, and fetal malformation were the leading predictors. Breech presentation was also a predictor, but breech delivery was not. This study showed that a large proportion of the cases of CP remain unexplained. Bejar et al. observed periventricular leukomalacia (PVL, multifocal necrosis of the white matter) on echo encephalography in utero. Their study suggested that there were prenatal antecedents of CP rather than intra-partum and post-natal factors [6]. Ultrasound of the brain is a useful noninvasive procedure that can demonstrate PVL and hemorrhagic brain lesions [7]. Magnetic resonance imaging (MRI) of the brain can also demonstrate hypoxic ischemic brain injury and can be used for the fetus, neonate, and infant [8].

Pathology

In general terms the areas of the brain which control movement are the motor cortex, basal ganglia, and cerebellum;

therefore, spastic CP is due to cerebral cortical damage, dyskinesia from basal ganglia damage, and ataxia from abnormalities of the cerebellum [2]. It is important to distinguish between spasticity, which is an increasing muscle contraction in response to stretch [9] and can be abolished by posterior root section, and rigidity, which is not affected by posterior root section. There are two clinical types of spasticity: phasic and tonic. In phasic spasticity the muscle does not produce a permanent contracture, whereas the tonic system is adapted to postural control and the muscle always resists stretching. This can induce shortening of the muscle and a joint contracture. In rigidity there is an involuntary, sustained contraction of the muscle, which is neither dependent on a stretch being applied to the muscle nor abolished by posterior root section. A clinical example of this is dystonic CP, which may be flexor or extensor. In clinical practice one sees "dynamic deformities" and an associated full range of movements under general anesthesia or slow and gentle examination. Although it is helpful to define tone patterns, many patients have a mixed neurological picture. Muscle weakness occurs in CP and may arise for several reasons, e.g., from underlying brain damage, immobility, and imbalance in musculotendinous lengths. The problem of muscle weakness in spastic conditions is increasingly gaining attention as part of maintenance of function. Reciprocal innervation of joint agonist and antagonist muscle groups provides a mechanism where one relaxes, while the other contracts. If only one group is weakened, a secondary and worse deformity may be produced by the unopposed action of the antagonist. Grading by the Medical Research Council (MRC) scale of strength in CP is difficult for the above reasons but is still useful clinically.

The brain develops despite the damage and adopts strategies to compensate for the deficits and to optimize function. The peripheral expression of the underlying central damage often changes as the patient grows. Compensatory mechanisms may, at first, be advantageous but later may result in secondary deformities. During growth, muscle has to keep pace with skeletal lengthening. In spastic paralysis there is relative shortening of the musculotendinous unit during growth and often little stretching of muscle during daily activities in some muscle groups. Ziv et al. have shown experimentally that muscle adds sarcomeres in response to constant stretch, but when muscles are spastic this mechanism does not occur [10]. Tardieu et al. believed that the major factor causing contracture was the maintenance of the muscle in a shortened position, either passively or by sustained contraction [11]. Deformity in CP may arise in several ways: as a result of brain damage, as an aberration of growth, and as a result of positional deformity. Compensatory mechanisms may produce deformity that results from management.

Deformities in CP may be mobile or fixed and arise from disorganized posture, balance, and movement.

Developmental delays cause retarded motor skills and the persistence of infantile reflexes. Delay in acquiring motor skills means that these appear later than normal and may be fewer than those in the normal child. There may also be variations and abnormal patterns in the motor skills that are subsequently acquired. There may be other reasons for motor delay such as visual handicap or learning difficulties. Immobility may be a result of multiple handicaps, blindness, and learning difficulties [12]. Postural mechanisms are an intrinsic part of motor skills and are linked to voluntary movement mechanisms. If equilibrium is poor, a child may not be able to initiate movement even though voluntary motion is possible. Retarded postural mechanisms may lead to lack of trunk and head control. Postural control and equilibrium dysfunction may be more pronounced if a potential compensation is impaired by a visual deficit. Abnormal reflexes may manifest as automatic stepping or the asymmetric tonic neck reflex, and recurring stimulation of abnormal reflexes may result in deformity. Abnormal postures develop from deformities as muscles shorten, or as a compensation to maintain equilibrium or its loss. They may also result from asymmetry of muscle function or from limb length inequality. Spasticity may also be used as a compensation, and the child relies on this to stand erect. Established contractures of one joint can have a subsequent effect on other joints, for example, a hip flexion contracture may cause equinus on the affected side. Isolated muscle groups are not spastic, but there is co-contraction of agonists and antagonists at any given joint. Usually it is the effect of the weaker antagonist that results in the deformity. This can be seen at the hip where abnormal forces cause joint subluxation or dislocation and the acetabulum then develops a deformity.

Physical Assessment

Static Examination

The patient lies supine on a couch, which can be replaced by mother's lap in young children. If the patient is positioned with the pelvis on the end of the couch, the legs are not supported. This position allows assessment of the range of motion of all joints of the lower extremities without moving the patient. The child can then be brought into the sitting position to observe head control, spinal deformity, and pelvic obliquity. In a walking child, the upper limbs are examined while the child sits. The assessment should include passive and active movements of the shoulder, elbow, wrist, and hand. Stance and gait need to be observed in a walker, appropriately undressed. Coordination and balance can be assessed by asking the child to stand or jump on one leg.

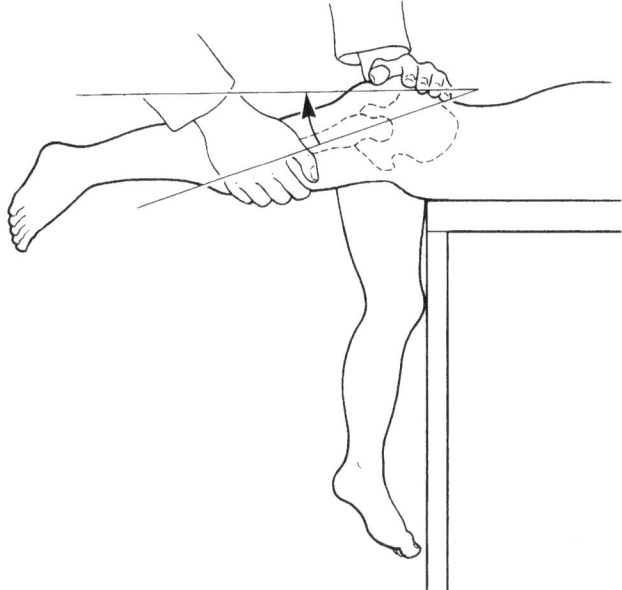

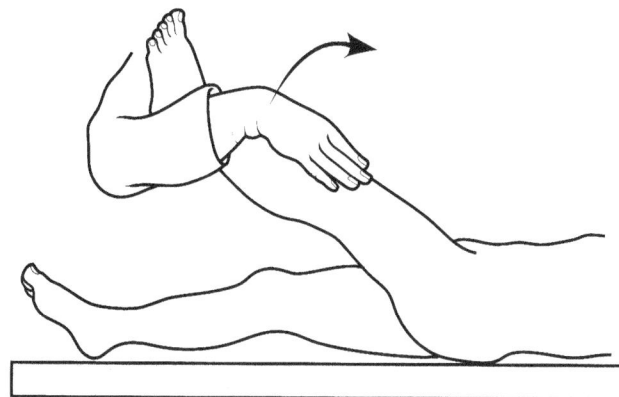

Fig. 6.2 Straight leg raising test to assess hamstring length

Fig. 6.1 Staheli hip extension test

Thomas's test is traditionally carried out and is accurate enough for clinical purposes but is less accurate than measuring hip flexion contractures as described by Staheli in the prone position (Fig. 6.1) [13]. The patient is placed so that the pelvis lies off the examining table and one hand is placed on the posterior superior spines, while the hip under examination is extended. The point of contracture is when the pelvis begins to tilt posteriorly. While supine, internal and external rotation and abduction and adduction can be measured. This is assessed with the hips in extension for a walker and with the hips in flexion for a nonwalker as these are the positions of function in these two circumstances. When assessing abduction and adduction it is essential to observe and palpate the anterior superior spines to allow an accurate assessment of the amount of abduction. If the spines are not visualized and felt, it is possible to show a "satisfactory" range of abduction when in reality on one side there may be only 5 or 10° of abduction and 30–40° on the opposite side. The knee is assessed for range of movement and capsular contracture. Straight leg raising assesses hamstring spasticity and contracture (Fig. 6.2). An alternative is to use the popliteal angle, which is found by flexing the hip to a right angle and extending the knee to the point of resistance. The popliteal angle lies between the vertical and the tibia at the point of resistance (Fig. 6.3).

The range of dorsiflexion of the ankle is measured with the heel held in inversion; this stabilizes the talonavicular joint and prevents lateral bow-stringing of the tendo-Achilles (escape valgus) when the heel is valgus thus producing a pseudo-correction. By holding the foot in varus, dorsiflexion of the mid-tarsal joints is prevented. In a varus deformity,

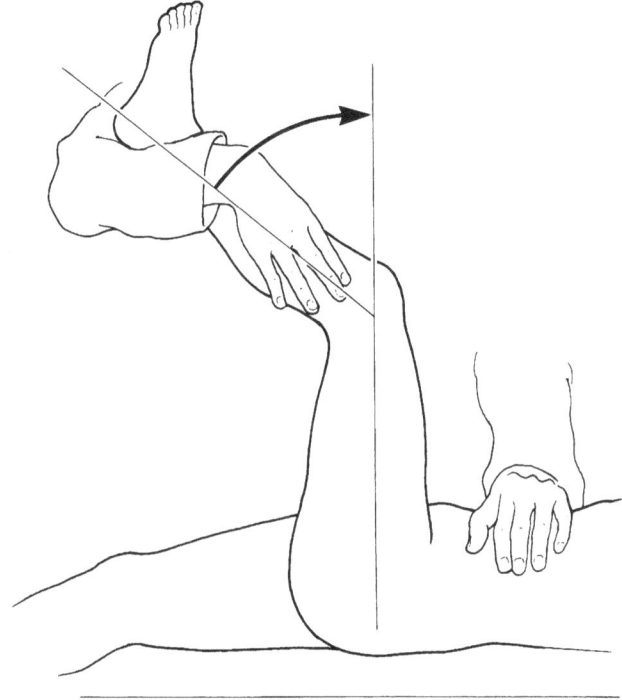

Fig. 6.3 Popliteal angle

however, the heel has to be kept in valgus. Traditionally Silverskiöld's test is used to differentiate between contracture of the gastrocnemius and soleus. The knee is flexed to 90° and the ankle/foot dorsiflexed, while the foot is held in inversion as far as possible, and an assessment is made of the foot–shank angle. This is then repeated with the knee fully extended. The amount of dorsiflexion when the inversion is released represents the overall mobility and instability of the hind- and mid-foot joints (Fig. 6.4). Subtalar and mid-tarsal movements can then be assessed along with toe deformities.

The patient is then moved up the couch and lies prone. Femoral anteversion is determined by palpation of the greater

Fig. 6.4 Dorsiflexion with the foot inverted (**a**) and everted (**b**)

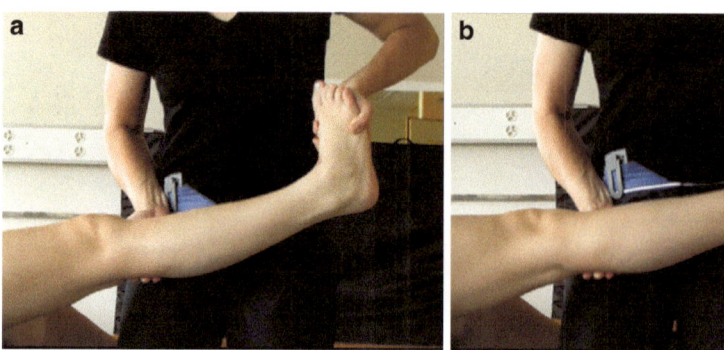

trochanter at its maximally prominent site and by measuring the angle between the tibia and the vertical [14]. The thigh–foot angle [15] is then assessed, giving an indirect clinical measurement of tibial torsion. The knee is flexed to 90° and the ankle is dorsiflexed into neutral, but without everting or inverting the foot. The relationship of the heel to the thigh is assessed visually or with a goniometer. The foot–thigh angle is invalid after hindfoot surgery. The examination so far will determine torsions between the femoral shaft and the calcaneus. There may be torsions within the foot itself. Because most patients have a mobile hindfoot, it may be more accurate to assess tibial torsion by measuring the angle between the transmalleolar axis and the femoral condyles or by using the footprint method [16]. The knee needs to be flexed to 90° for this measurement.

Traditional stretch tests are inaccurate in CP and have limited specificity. The Duncan Ely test (rectus stretch test) also generates action potentials in iliopsoas [17] and the Thomas test generates similar electrical activity in rectus and iliopsoas. Phelp's (gracilis) test and straight leg raising induce the same amount of electrical activity in the medial hamstrings. The specificity of Silverskiöld's test has been questioned by Perry et al., because on electromyography both gastrocnemius and soleus showed increased action potentials irrespective of the position of the knee [18].

Evaluation of Gait

Walking is a complex activity, and events occur in the coronal, sagittal, and transverse planes. Descriptions of the gait cycle have been traditionally made in the sagittal plane. The goals of gait are stability and progression. The prerequisites are stance phase stability, swing phase clearance, foot preposition in terminal swing, adequate step length, and energy conservation [19]. The upper body must be supported in both double and single supports and may be challenged by two factors: first by body weight and second by the alterations of the body segments during walking.

Smooth progression depends upon the maintenance of forward velocity, clearance of the leg in swing, and absorption of energy before and at foot contact. During single support there are two main progressional forces: first, there is the input of energy to stabilize the lower limb and to assist the upward and forward motion of the hip and upper body. This is then followed by a controlled and downward fall of the body from a high point and represents the conversion of potential to kinetic energy assisted by gravity.

Visual observation of gait is used traditionally to assess aberrations in walking patterns. In practice it is difficult to perform this accurately when there are abnormalities at several anatomical levels—trunk, pelvis, hip, knee, ankle, and foot, and in three planes. One effective way of improving gait observation is to employ video recordings and a freeze-frame playback facility or to use a visual gait score such as the Edinburgh Gait score [20]. Gait analysis (Chapter 26) has become an important investigative tool in CP and in some centers is regarded as essential before surgery for the walker. Gait analysis certainly provides a means of objective audit after intervention, but not all have access to this complex type of investigation. A comprehensive gait evaluation in CP would include kinematics, kinetics, energy consumption, and dynamic electromyography (EMG).

Although ungainly, abnormal walking patterns may represent the most efficient method of progression for the child and result from a variety of factors. The walking pattern may be a compensation for deficient control of equilibrium, joint contracture, or muscle spasticity. Many children with CP are effectively in a state of "collapse" and cannot support their body weight on one leg thus walking rapidly to avoid falling over. Patients with CP may also have an excessive forward lean of the trunk when walking to control extension at the knee. The common pattern in hemiplegia and diplegia is internal rotation, flexion, and adduction of the hip (Fig. 6.5). There may also be flexion of the knee and an equinus posture of the ankle. The knee may extend fully passively but may tend to be in valgus when walking, although there may not be a fixed valgus deformity. Secondary deformities may ensue, such as external tibial torsion distal to

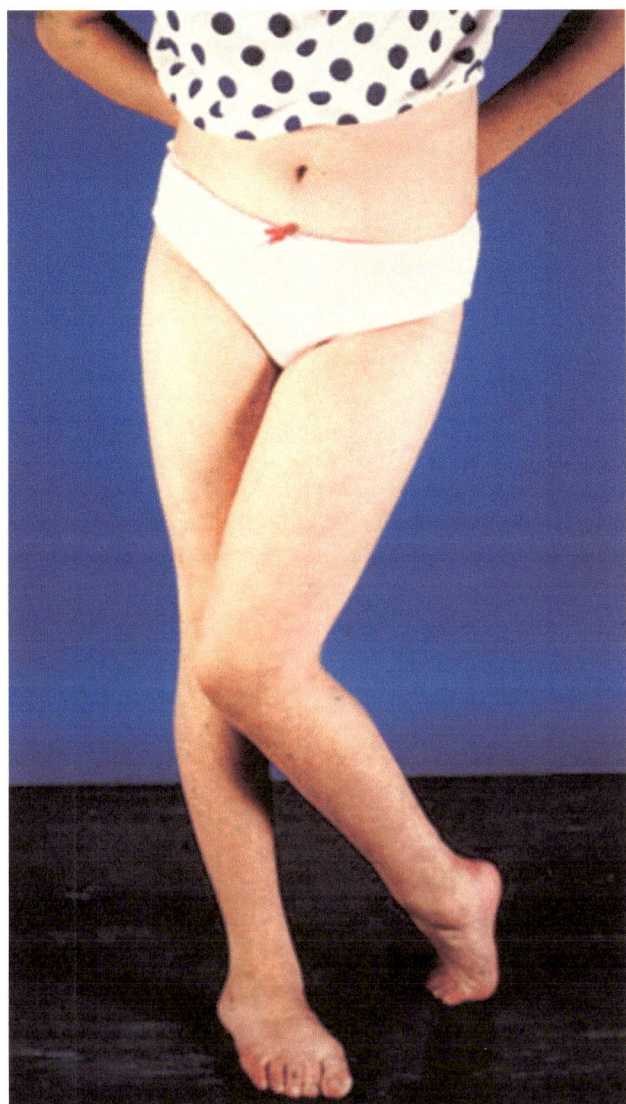

Fig. 6.5 Typical posture of adduction and internal rotation at the hip, and flexion at the knee and ankle

excessive internal femoral torsion. A valgus calcaneus and pes valgus are common associated deformities.

One way of compensating for muscle weakness is to control the center of gravity to unload a weak muscle. For example, in Duchenne type of gait pattern (lateral trunk lean toward the affected hip) the lateralization of the center of mass minimizes the commonly present external hip adduction moment which requires hip abductor activity to avoid contralateral pelvic drop. Similarly, knee extension can be controlled by forward lean of the trunk which reduces the load on the knee extensors.

The aim of clinical examination and gait analysis is to define a list of biomechanical problems apart from the neurological disorder, having considered muscle length, strength, bony lever arms, and alignment.

Principles and Aims of Management

In general, the shape of the locomotor system depends upon function, which depends upon use. This explains why a joint can lose motion if its range is not used. One aim in the management of patients with CP therefore involves control of posture and daily activities, during which the available range of joint movement and muscle length should be used.

It is important to distinguish between disturbances of function due to the underlying condition, useful adaptations, which may look abnormal, and functional difficulties secondary to deformity. Compromises may have to be made between the balance of benefit from an intervention and the disadvantages. For example, standing with the knees bent places a load on the quadriceps, which is tiring. Straightening the knees can solve this stance phase problem for the patient but may cause difficulties in the swing phase of gait.

Dynamic instability, or lever arm dysfunction, is a major factor interfering with movement and can result in bony deformity and joint dislocations. For example, in diplegia many patients have increased femoral anteversion and initially walk on tiptoe. Pes valgus then commonly develops and the foot becomes externally rotated with respect to the tibia but is also functionally plantigrade. External tibial torsion may then develop as a consequence of the pes valgus and increased femoral anteversion produces the so-called miserable malalignment. Joints can be stabilized with orthoses or by arthrodesis. Absolute stability at a given joint may be a disadvantage in the longer term and can remove some compensatory movement for a deformity at a more proximal level.

Some patients with CP appear to have strong muscles but spasticity often masks an underlying muscle weakness. The imbalance of muscle action across a joint may be managed by lengthening or weakening the agonist to restore the imbalance between agonist and antagonist. Force and length are related to each other physiologically. Lengthening results in a reduction of force and is used to gain length or to reduce force. Muscle tension may decrease after tendon transfers and a reduction of force is seen as a secondary phenomenon. Thus reduction of muscle force is a regular consequence of nonoperative and operative managements. The effect is transient after casting or aponeurotic (intramuscular) lengthening [21] but longer lasting after tendon lengthening [21–23]. Force reduction may give the impression of being advantageous, because spasticity seems to be reduced. In reality, however, the output from the central nervous system remains unchanged although spasticity may be less noticeable due to the decrease in muscle force. The advantage of reduction of spasticity may be counteracted by the disadvantage of muscle weakness for postural control and function. Hence muscle strengthening exercises may help to improve function despite concerns about possibly increasing spasticity [24]. The aims of management have to take into account the overall function of the patient and the existence of a deformity which does not necessarily merit treatment.

Orthotic Management

The general aims of orthoses are to provide stability in dynamic and static conditions, to control the position and shape of body segments, and to guide motion. Hence they are used to control function, to correct and prevent deformities, and to substitute for missing muscle activity and strength. They can be used as aids worn during function or as positional devices such as night splints. However, as function is impaired by malposition of joints, instability, and deformity, the efficacy of functional orthoses is generally superior to a positional device. Orthoses should only be used if benefits outweigh disadvantages.

Ankle–foot orthoses (AFOs) may be prescribed for several reasons: to maintain posture, to prevent deformity, and to obtain a biomechanical effect. They may be used for walkers and nonwalkers. The manufacture of an orthosis depends upon an accurate, positive plaster cast of the child's foot and calf, from which a lightweight thermoplastic splint is manufactured. Apart from static functions, such as preventing deformity and maintaining posture, the orthosis can be used to alter the biomechanical forces acting upon joints.

When the foot is applied to the ground, an equal and opposite ground reaction force is generated in response to this load (Newton's third law). The ground reaction force has magnitude in three directions and can be measured with a force plate (see Chapter 26). Knowledge of the orientation of the vertical component of the ground reaction force to any given joint is helpful when changing orthotic prescription. In the case of the child with crouch gait, where the vertical component of the ground reaction force is flexor in relation to the knee, the goal is to change the direction of the ground reaction force to pass through the knee joint. During normal walking there is a smooth progression of the ground reaction force origin from the heel at foot contact to the metatarsal heads at foot-off. In the case of crouch gait, the origin of the ground reaction force remains at the heel throughout stance, and forward progression of the upper body over the stationary foot occurs by an excessive amount of tibial progression over the foot, resulting in knee flexion. The AFO prevents excessive tibial progression in relation to the foot (Fig. 6.6) [25]. This then re-orientates the vertical component of the ground reaction force so that it passes through or near to the knee joint center, and thus the patient walks in a more upright posture. AFOs are a powerful tool, not just a piece of plastic, and can have dramatic and reversible effects upon

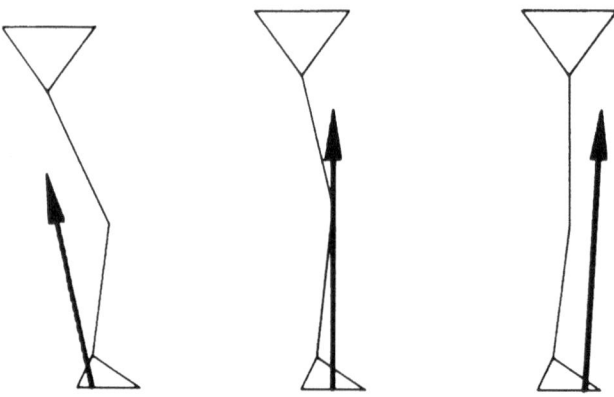

Fig. 6.6 Effect of an ankle–foot orthosis on crouch gait. Diagrammatic representation of the pelvis, thigh, shank, and foot in the sagittal plane. The arrow indicates the vertical component of the ground reaction force

the biomechanics of gait as well as standing posture. They are usually worn in normal shoewear, and these shoes always have a slight heel raise. The shank axis needs to be perpendicular to the floor as in normal standing and the height of the heel on the shoe needs to be taken into account when setting the foot–shank angle of the AFO. A little plantar flexion (or equinus) of about 5° is often left in the AFO so that the AFO–shoewear combination gives a satisfactory orientation of the shank to the vertical. If this is not taken into account, standing is comparable to standing in a ski boot with a slight anterior tilt.

Orthoses can be used to modify different phases of the gait cycle. The goal of foot contact is to bring the heel down first on the ground. An orthosis can be used here to control a drop foot, to permit heel contact rather than toe contact with the ground, or to control varus or valgus alignment of the foot. An analogy would be an aircraft landing on its main wheels, not on the nose wheel. During the loading response the orthosis can substitute for pretibial muscle function and prevent excessive inversion or eversion, and an orthotic modification for this phase would be the provision of a solid ankle cushion heel. The aircraft analogy in this case would be to prevent the wheels buckling on landing. During the first phase of single support the goal is tibial progression over the stationary foot with control of the ground reaction force in relation to the hip and knee. Here excessive tibial progression can be prevented by the use of an AFO or a floor reaction orthosis. An externally applied rocker to the shoe may also allow a smoother progression of the foot along the floor. In terminal stance the goal is to provide acceleration of the limb before pre-swing. There is no orthotic solution for problems in this phase of the gait cycle at present. In CP the main use of the AFO is to substitute for tibialis anterior and gastrocnemius and soleus activity. In swing the prerequisites are limb clearance and step length so in this phase the orthosis will compensate for a foot drop and preposition the foot in terminal swing. Orthoses should not interfere with knee motion. These various demands are best achieved with mobile, flexible orthoses, which improve gait more than rigid ones in the walker [26]. Resting orthoses may be used at night to minimize future deformity or to stretch contracted muscles. However, stretching can be an uncomfortable sensation and interfere with sleep. For this reason, orthoses are often poorly tolerated at night or are tolerated if no stretch is applied. The orthosis is then no longer functioning as intended.

A knee–ankle–foot orthosis (KAFO) may be indicated to stretch short hamstrings. This orthosis is applied during rest, but not at night, under full tension for 1–2 h during the daytime. The KAFO can also be used post-operatively and has the advantage over plaster of being removable. This helps to prevent neurological compromise or skin pressure problems. There is increasing interest in using dynamic orthoses in the management of knee contractures [27] but their efficacy in the longer term is unknown.

Thoraco-lumbar orthoses are used to control trunk posture in the nonwalker but only have a minor effect, compared to surgery, on the natural history of spinal deformity progression in neuromuscular scoliosis which is independent of the adolescent growth spurt [28, 29]. Early onset of conservative treatment and good correction by the brace are essential factors for a good postural effect [28]. Progress is monitored by radiographs taken with the patient erect in the brace (Fig. 6.7). If used in a walker who has a spinal deformity, the brace should allow some spinal motion when this is being

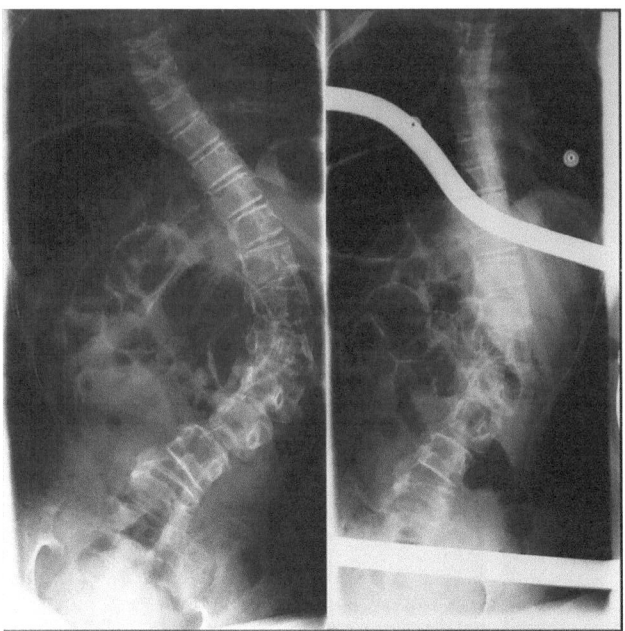

Fig. 6.7 Spinal alignment in and out of a thoraco-lumbar-sacral orthosis

used to compensate for a stiff leg gait. Stabilizing the spine in a nonwalker can substitute for weak paraspinal muscles, thereby improving head control and hand function.

Surgery

Abnormal tone, muscle imbalance, contractures, and bony deformity are amenable to surgery. Bony deformities and contractures are typical indications for orthopaedic intervention. Muscle balancing procedures, however, can be done for an imbalance of strength or length but muscle strength will be diminished as a result of muscle or tendon lengthening, which may not always benefit the patient. Problems resulting from excessive tone, rather than muscle shortening, require tone management. The fundamental injury to the central nervous system, namely loss of selective control and persistent reflex activity, is incurable. There are two important steps in assessing a patient for surgery: clinical examination and assessment of gait in the walking patient. An examination under anesthesia can be carried out separately but is usually unnecessary if a gentle and slow technique of assessment is used during clinical examination.

Orthopaedic operations may involve muscle or tendon lengthening (Fig. 6.8), tendon transfers, tenotomy, bony operations to improve rotational problems or to relocate joints, and neurectomy. Although surgery to the muscles and tendons will weaken the muscle, soft tissue surgery alone will not correct a fixed skeletal deformity. There is a trend now to perform surgery at one stage where possible, and operations in the walking child can be designed for both swing and stance phase problems. In the presence of mobile deformity the surgeon should think of balancing procedures around joints, whereas rotational and fixed bony deformities require bony surgery.

Tone Management

Selective posterior rhizotomy for reduction in spasticity has been popularized by Peacock et al. [30]. Its objective is to obtain a better balance between facilitatory and inhibitory control of the anterior horn cells. They have reported encouraging data in predominantly spastic diplegic patients where spasticity of muscle was reduced even to the point of flaccidity. The procedure entails selective sectioning of approximately one-quarter to one-half of the L2-S1 nerve rootlets that demonstrate abnormal responses to electrical stimulation at the time of surgery. This does not abolish primitive motor reflexes or fixed contractures of musculotendinous units or joints.

The ideal patient for rhizotomy is a walking spastic diplegic who has minimal fixed contractures, but the approach may also be helpful for the nonwalker with total body involvement. Other favorable criteria include prematurity, pure spasticity, good trunk control and strength, minimal contractures, motivation, and the availability of physiotherapy. Poor indicators are hemiplegia, weakness of antigravity muscles, rigidity, dystonia, athetosis, marked flexion contractures, and fixed spinal deformity [31]. One concern after rhizotomy is the possibility of producing later spinal deformity, which could result from post-operative hypotonia and the laminectomy. Spiegel et al. found that after selective dorsal rhizotomy (SDR) using a laminoplasty technique, 12% of children developed a spondylolisthesis and 17% a scoliosis [32]. Greene et al. reported rapid progression of hip subluxation in six patients during the year after SDR, which was explained by the reduced sensory input from the joint, necessary for dynamic control [33]. Normally the L1 root is preserved, so the hip flexors may not be as denervated as their antagonists, thus predisposing to dysplasia. Steinbok has confirmed the benefits of SDR in spastic diplegia and a more limited role in spastic quadriplegia [34]. He found very strong evidence that SDR results in improvements in lower limb spasticity, an increase in the range of movement in the lower limb joints, and either no change or improvement in lower limb strength. There is moderate certainty that improvements in impairment are maintained up to 5 years after SDR and some weaker evidence that the improvements are maintained in the longer term. There is good evidence from prospective case series that there are improvements in self-care and performance of activities of daily living after SDR. The advantage of SDR is that the procedure is definitive, and the patient is not dependent upon lifelong medication as is the case with a baclofen pump [35]. The functional benefit of SDR seems to be even greater than after multi-level surgery [36]. SDR, however, may have significant and persistent complications such as muscle weakness and sphincter incontinence.

Oral baclofen has been used for many years to reduce spasticity, but often therapeutic doses cause drowsiness and excessive drooling. The intrathecal route delivers the drug close to its site of action at the spinal cord and much lower doses are needed to produce a therapeutic tone-reducing effect. The pump is inserted in the subcutaneous or subfascial layer of the anterior abdominal wall and a catheter is routed subcutaneously into the intrathecal space. Intrathecal baclofen (ITB) reduces tone and pain thus easing care and improving function [37, 38]. The main advantages of ITB are that the dose can be tailored to the patient's requirements and that the effects are reversible. The main disadvantages are a 5% risk of infection, the need to renew the batteries of the pump after about 5 years, and the fact that the therapy is not definitive. Albright has concluded that ITB is an effective treatment for children with hypertonicity secondary to spasticity and dystonia and often results in dramatic improvements in quality of life and in easier care [39]. In spite of the complications, most families and patients ask to continue ITB therapy at the end of pump battery life. There has been concern about the risk of spinal curvature increasing after ITB. For example, Ginsburg and Lauder found a significant increase in spinal deformity if trunk control was reduced [40]. However, Senaran et al. have shown that the procedure did not have a significant effect on spinal curve progression, pelvic obliquity, or the incidence of scoliosis when compared with an age, gender, and GMFCS score-matched control group of patients with spastic CP without an ITB pump [41].

Intramuscular botulinum toxin A is another drug which has gained increasing importance in the management of spastic muscles. The toxin irreversibly blocks the release of acetyl choline from the neuromuscular end plate causing a flaccid paralysis of the muscle but muscle activity recovers as new end plates form after about 3 months. Cosgrove et al. reported a beneficial effect on muscle growth in spastic mice [42]. Good, but often temporary, functional improvements

Fig. 6.8 Techniques of musculotendinous lengthening. (**a**) Z-lengthening, (**b**) intramuscular tendon lengthening, and (**c**) aponeurotomy

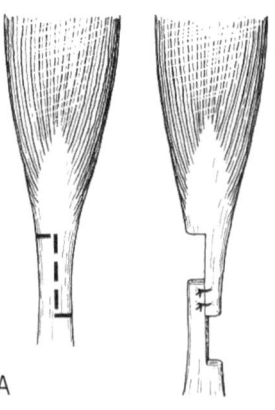
A

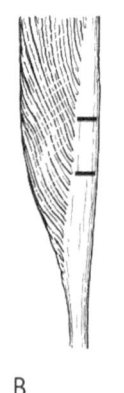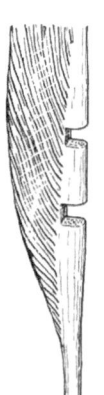
B

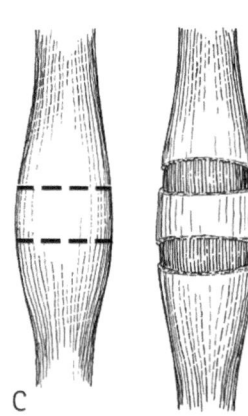
C

Fig. 6.9 Before and after soft tissue releases for seating and perineal access

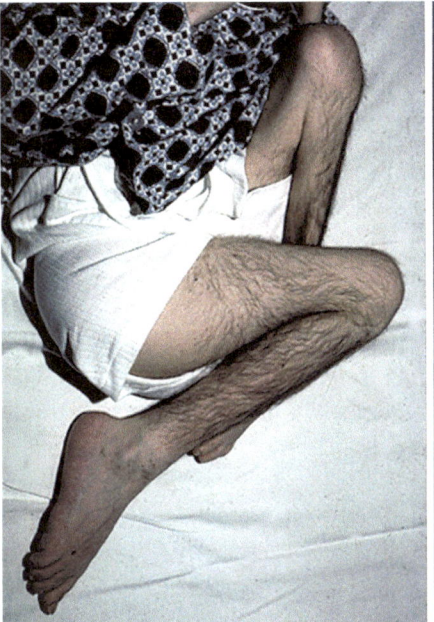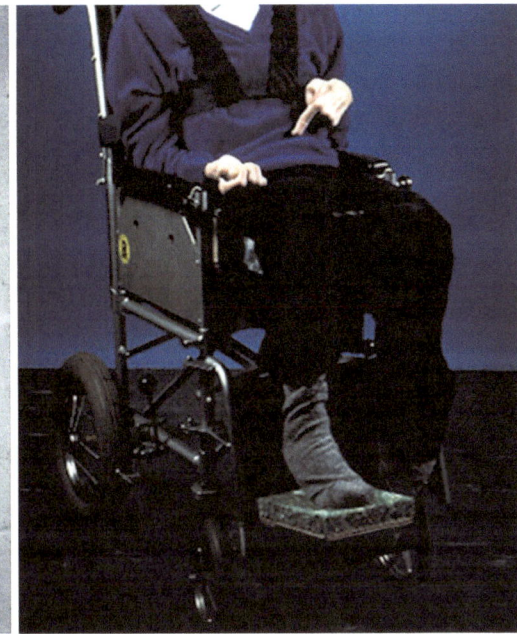

are seen in younger patients where muscle tone is the dominant problem [43]. Molenaers et al. found that botulinum toxin A treatment delayed and reduced the frequency of surgical procedures in children with CP who were able to walk [44]. Target muscles can be identified from gait analysis and apart from delaying the need for muscle surgery the botulinum toxin A can also give an indication of the possible functional outcome of muscle surgery by weakening the target muscle. The injections are often combined with casting and/or physiotherapy to stretch a shortened muscle. Botulinum toxin A injections have also been used in post-operative management following multi-level surgery in CP.

Surgery to a muscle may also reduce spasticity. Tardieu et al. have shown that tendon lengthening results in a persistent loss of muscle strength [23]. However, muscle strength is only temporarily reduced after intramuscular or aponeurotic lengthening procedures [21] (Fig. 6.8).

Surgery for the Nonwalker

It can be very difficult to assess a patient's functional ability in the presence of severe impairment. Often the clinician has to rely on the parents, carers, or therapists for further information. Assessment of "hip" pain can be difficult as, in the total body-involved patient, gastrointestinal pain can present as pain in the hip region. Severe handicap of itself should not prevent treatment.

The major cause of restricted function in severely affected patients is the lack of coordination and muscle control. One

of the major goals for a nonwalker is to acquire the ability to transfer either independently or with a helper. Any intervention which may interfere with lower limb joint stability, for example, proximal femoral resection for hip dislocation, may be disadvantageous for the patient who is capable of an assisted transfer. Management of severe secondary deformities should not affect existing function.

Goals in this group are different from those in walking patients, and mostly orientated toward a pain-free existence, balanced seating or, if the patient is capable of transfers, plantigrade feet, and the reduction of knee and hip flexion contractures. Adduction deformities of the hip can be particularly troublesome for seating and nappy (diaper) changing (Fig. 6.9).

Spinal Deformities

The cause of spinal deformity is the lack of dynamic muscle control to counteract the deforming force of gravity. The greater the deformity, the greater the lever arm for the deforming force and the faster the progression. Thoracolumbar orthoses can stabilize the trunk in an upright position and reduce progression of the spinal deformity, although they are less efficient than surgery [28]. They may also be used to assist trunk control during feeding or to provide trunk stability for arm function.

The spine should not be viewed in isolation. Hip dislocation, subluxation, and pelvic obliquity often coexist with scoliosis. James found that muscle release operations beneath the iliac crest did not alter the scoliosis [45], and Lonstein and Beck failed to find any association between hip dislocation, pelvic obliquity, and scoliosis in CP; the scoliosis developed regardless of the pelvic position [46]. Although single and double thoraco-lumbar curves occur in CP, the single C-type curve occurs more frequently in the total body-involved patient, who usually has absent truncal equilibrium reactions and pelvic obliquity. Curve progression is inevitable, and Madigan and Wallace found that the greatest progression was in the most severely involved groups [47]. Curves continue to progress even after skeletal maturity [48]. If the curve is progressive and threatens the child's ability to sit in spite of wheelchair modifications and bracing, surgical stabilization of the spine should be considered. Recently there has been greater interest in performing spinal fusion, even in the severely handicapped child who is a permanent wheelchair user. Indications include a severe sagittal plane deformity, loss of sitting ability or balance, back pain and pain from impingement of the ribs against the hemipelvis, and inefficacy of a spinal brace. Surgical stabilization of the spine can either extend to the sacrum, thereby removing any possibility of compensatory movement, or leave the L5-S1 segment free, allowing some mobility but the risk of subsequent lumbosacral pain. If there is fixed pelvic obliquity, the fusion should extend to the sacrum. This is major surgery, and severe learning difficulties or handicap may present a quandary for the parents or caregivers. Technical details of this type of surgery using a unit rod have been reported by Dabney et al. [49]. Studies have confirmed parental and carer satisfaction with spinal stabilization but functional benefits for the individual have been less easy to define [29, 50]. However, relieving the patient of discomfort due to pelvic obliquity and rib impingement on the iliac crest is likely to be an advantage and the patient with a straighter spine is easier to nurse and seat.

Kyphosis is also seen and usually begins as a postural problem in patients who have poor trunk and head control. It is flexible initially but can become fixed during subsequent growth. Severe kyphosis is a disabling deformity. In severe cases surgical correction including anterior release and posterior correction and fusion is indicated. Hyperlordosis is usually indicative of hip flexion contractures. The sacrum becomes almost horizontal and back pain often ensues. Because severe and persistent hyperlordosis can become painful a persistent lordotic posture should be avoided.

The Hip

The windswept deformity (adduction contracture and increased internal rotation of one hip and displacement of the other hip in abduction and external rotation) is a typical finding in the nonwalker and causes difficulties with perineal hygiene and seating. The incidence of hip displacement varies but in a recent study the risk of displacement was found to be directly related to gross motor function as graded by the GMFCS [51]. The risk was 0% in children in GMFCS level I and 90% in GMFCS level V. Bracing is not effective in spastic hip displacement. Graham et al. studied the combined effect of intramuscular injection of botulinum toxin A and abduction hip bracing in the management of spastic hip displacement in a randomized trial and found that progressive hip displacement continued to occur in the treatment group. They did not recommend this treatment [52].

In the absence of hip flexion contracture, myotomy of gracilis and an intramuscular adductor tenotomy of adductor longus are usually sufficient, provided symmetry of abduction can be obtained (Fig. 6.10). A more extensive procedure, including an anterior obturator neurectomy or more extensive myotomy, should not be carried out as an extreme abduction deformity and loss of dynamic control of the hip may result and cannot be remedied. The latter is especially a concern for patients who are almost, or just able, to transfer as this capability will be lost after excessive adductor lengthening.

The cause of hip dislocation in CP is not clear, but some assumptions are possible. The hip is, as a rule, normal at birth but acetabular enlargement gradually ensues as result of lack of dynamic control and may result in dislocation. Another factor may be positioning [2, 53] and many children with severe CP rest in the same position particularly at night, such as side-lying where one hip remains in adduction. The role of spasticity remains unclear, but is probably

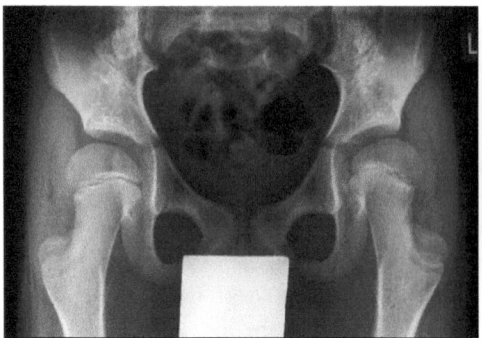 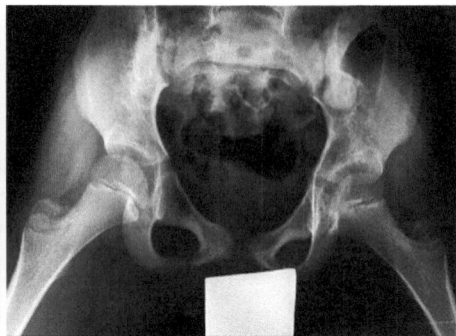

Fig. 6.10 Uncovering of the femoral heads improved with abduction of the hips

Fig. 6.11 Reimer's migration index is the part of the femoral epiphysis extending beyond Perkins' line (P) expressed as a percentage of the entire width of the epiphysis measured in the horizontal plane

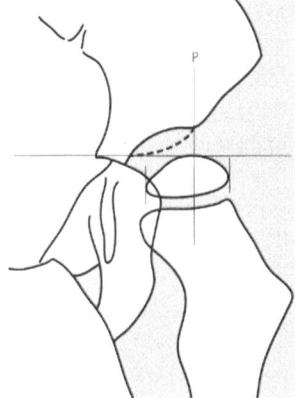

overestimated, because hip dislocations occur in hypotonic as well as hypertonic conditions. Another factor may be impaired proprioception which results in inadequate muscle control [4].

Clinical signs are unreliable in making the diagnosis of a hip dislocation, as contractures are common and restrict motion. The diagnosis is made from radiographs. Although standard radiological criteria can be used, a critical assessment of the patient and radiograph is important as geometric indices such as the Reimer's migration index [54] (Fig. 6.11) or the Wiberg center–edge angle depend upon the position of the joint at any given moment and are influenced by rotation and adduction. Faraj and colleagues have recently questioned the reliability of Reimers' index for clinical purposes as they found significant inter-observer errors that could be outside clinical acceptability [55]. A better early indicator is the lateral acetabular edge [56]. A progressive convexity indicates excessive pressure from the femoral head against the acetabular edge and progression to femoral head displacement with time. In this instance the risk of dislocation remains despite normal geometry.

Arthrographic findings show that progressive deformation of the cartilaginous acetabulum and femoral head occurs in some cases before obvious hip instability [57]. The hip develops a typical deformity during this dislocation process which consists of a unidirectional enlargement of the acetabulum, unidirectional joint instability, and then joint decentering. On the femoral side increased anteversion and/or valgus and muscle contractures are seen [58]. As 91% of the hips dislocate cranio-laterally this deformity is seen on antero-posterior radiographs of the pelvis. Other directions of dislocation exist, however (anterior 8%, posterior 1%), and are sometimes only visible on 3D-computed tomography (CT) scans.

Treatment for hip dislocation is indicated for three reasons: instability, which cannot be controlled by the patient; restriction of motion, which predisposes to pathological fractures; and pain, which may already be present in mild subluxations [59, 60]. There is controversy, however, as to whether a dislocated hip is painful, but Cooperman et al. suggested that 50% of a small group of institutionalized patients with CP complained of pain in the dislocated hip [61]. They concluded that a dislocation should be reduced. Noonan et al. found that the incidence of hip pain was low and not associated with hip displacement or osteoarthritis in their study of 77 adults with CP [62]. They recommended that surgical treatment of the hip in severely affected patients should be based upon the presence of pain or contractures and not on radiographic signs of hip displacement or osteoarthritis. In many centers children with severe CP have a hip surveillance program consisting of an annual pelvic radiograph after the age of 5 until skeletal maturity [63]. Under the age of 5 years progressive lateral displacement of the head is managed in some centers by adductor longus intramuscular tenotomy, gracilis myotomy, and psoas tenotomy. This is only likely to be effective in the longer term if hip abduction can be maintained. Progressive uncovering of the femoral head requires the addition of varus derotation osteotomy [64]. A varus osteotomy of the femur has the same effect as passive hip abduction but has the advantage that its effect is independent of passive movement. The femoral deformity is either excessive anteversion or valgus, or both. It should be remembered that coxa valga is often a radiographic artefact due to femoral torsion, so that a corrected view of the proximal femur should be obtained. An antero-posterior radiograph with the femur in internal rotation to neutralize anteversion is a prerequisite to show the true femoral pathology and the neck–shaft angle. The aim of surgery is to restore the neck–shaft angle and an AO blade plate provides excellent fixation for this purpose. Significant re-operation rates have been reported after early soft tissue or proximal femoral procedures when performed at an average age of 4 years, as acetabular remodeling did not reliably occur post-operatively [65]. In practice many nonwalking children with CP present to the orthopaedic surgeon with established radiological signs of hip displacement. Where there is acetabular dysplasia or a dislocation, the femoral osteotomy needs to be supplemented by an acetabular procedure such as a Pemberton [66] or Dega pelvic osteotomy [67]. These procedures bend down the elongated part of the acetabulum over the reduced femoral head. It is also possible to perform a Dega osteotomy after closure of the triradiate cartilage in patients with severe CP as the pelvic bone is often osteoporotic [68]. Procedures to redirect the acetabulum or to enlarge femoral head cover are less effective and are indicated for other acetabular pathologies. An open reduction of the hip is not always necessary but when needed should include resection of the ligamentum teres and division of the transverse acetabular ligament. Sufficient shortening of the femur at the time of femoral osteotomy is most important to lengthen, relatively, the contracted muscles and to avoid pressure on the femoral head; additional soft tissue procedures are rarely necessary. This complex operation has a success rate of about 95% in experienced hands for lateral or posterior dislocations, but for anterior dislocation there is a failure rate of up to 30%. Even severe deformity of the femoral head is not necessarily a contraindication to reduction since the risk of subsequent arthritis appears to be small. If the femoral head is unreconstructable, there is a choice of procedures to obtain reasonable abduction. The demand on the hip in these severely handicapped patients is low and osteoarthritic changes seen radiologically can remain asymptomatic for many years. A subtrochanteric abduction osteotomy can be carried out which will give sufficient abduction for perineal hygiene and seating [69]. Proximal femoral resection has been plagued by ectopic bone formation but may be prevented by the technique of interposition arthroplasty described by Castle and Schneider using the gluteus medius and minimus and vastus lateralis between the resected femur and the acetabulum [70].

The Knee

In the nonwalker the goals of treatment for the knee are to obtain a comfortable posture when sitting in a chair, lying in bed, and standing in a standing frame, if such a device is used. Excessive knee flexion causes skin problems on the edge of the chair. Fractional hamstring lengthening rarely brings complete correction but may be enough to improve hamstring length sufficiently. If the result is insufficient, a closing wedge supracondylar extension osteotomy can be added. This will not give the patient any further range of motion but will change the arc of available movement to a more useful one.

Foot and Ankle Deformity

In the nonwalker, the goals are a well-shaped foot for shoewear, for the foot to rest on the footplate of the wheelchair, and for it to be plantigrade when standing in a standing frame. Severe equinus is undesirable. Fixed bony deformity may have to be corrected by bony surgery. Joint fusions are well tolerated and provide long-lasting results, whereas there is a high risk of the deformity recurring after soft tissue procedures alone.

Surgery for the Walker

One prerequisite for normal gait is to be able to use as little energy or muscle force as possible, compatible with efficient locomotion. Ideally the ground reaction force should pass behind the hip joint center and in front of the knee joint center thereby creating passive external knee and hip extensor moments. Mild hyperextension at the knee and hip helps to stabilize these joints in stance as the patient can use their ligaments and capsule as a "backstop" to counteract the external extension moment. The position of the shank relative to the floor is critical for the triceps surae to control the ground reaction forces with respect to the proximal joints. The position of the foot relative to the floor is less critical, but to increase stability the heel should contact the floor. This can be achieved by adding a heel raise to the shoe if there is equinus. During swing the leg must shorten functionally to pass the opposite leg. The knee must extend again in terminal swing before the foot next contacts the ground.

There are surgical solutions for both the stance and the swing phases of gait. Correction of deformities should be considered in the sagittal, coronal, and transverse planes. Only a small percentage of patients with total body involvement are mobile, and the following section relates mainly to those with diplegia and hemiplegia. Multi-level surgery based on pre- and post-operative gait analysis has been shown to be effective for the walking child with CP [71, 72] and health-related quality of life outcomes also improve post-operatively [73].

The Hip

Loss of extension of the hip is a problem and will also influence the position of the knee and ankle. It is of less importance, however, if the patient can only walk with aids, resulting in a flexed position of the trunk when standing or walking. Although intramuscular psoas tenotomy has been advocated this has to be balanced against the possible risk of post-operative hip flexor weakness that could affect forward propulsion of the lower limb. Preservation of hip flexor strength is important for patients with CP and there is now a trend away from psoas lengthening. Adduction contracture of the hip may be manifested by short stride length, approximation of the knees, and, in severe cases, scissoring. In walking patients who have a functional adduction deformity shown by gait analysis, intramuscular adductor longus tenotomy and gracilis myotomy are the procedures of choice, but it is important to be sure that the "adducted" posture of the knees is not due to internal femoral rotation. If there is asymmetry of abduction, the adductor longus tendon and gracilis may be tenotomized on one side and the gracilis only on the other. Anterior branch obturator neurectomy is contraindicated in the walking patient because the adductor brevis muscle, a hip stabilizer, is denervated.

Internal rotation deformity can be corrected by derotation femoral osteotomy. Biomechanical analysis has shown that the level of correction, subtrochanteric or supracondylar, does not affect the end result [74]. The site of osteotomy is chosen with regard to concomitant procedures such as correction of a knee flexion contracture or femoral neck–shaft angle. A blade plate can be used either proximally or distally and gives excellent fixation. In general it is better to delay derotation osteotomy until 7 or 8 years of age as femoral torsion does not change significantly in children after the age of 9 and may recur if performed in younger children [75, 76]. When assessing rotational deformity in the leg, it is important that a compensatory external tibial torsion is not made more obvious after femoral derotation osteotomy and is recognized and corrected at the same time.

Dislocated or subluxed hip joints are treated as in the nonwalker by joint reconstruction including open reduction, if necessary, femoral and pelvic osteotomy, and, rarely, additional soft tissue procedures. It is preferable to shorten the femur enough to reduce pressure within the joint and hence avoid femoral head necrosis than to preserve leg length. Residual leg length discrepancy can be corrected toward skeletal maturity by a contralateral epiphysiodesis at the knee.

Internal rotation is a common deformity in walkers but is not necessarily functionally disabling. Patients may have difficulties in controlling their legs which may give way and flex at the knees. An internally rotated position of the lower limbs places the flexed legs under the center of mass and requires less compensatory movement to rebalance the trunk. In external rotation, however, the patient must still position the trunk over the lower limb to attempt to align the center of mass, which often results in a Duchenne type of gait pattern (lateral lean of the trunk toward the stance lower limb). For this reason there is now a trend toward leaving some residual internal rotation of not more than 10° when improving internal femoral rotation surgically.

The Knee

There may be extension or flexion deformities at the knee. A flexed knee posture may have several causes, for example, spasticity of the hamstrings, weakness of the quadriceps, a hip flexion contracture, spasticity of the gastrocnemius, or a combination of these factors. The joints above and below the knee should be examined as the knee should not be considered in isolation. Fractional lengthening of the medial hamstrings is the procedure of choice if the hamstrings are to be lengthened and allows some choice over the degree of lengthening. The problem with co-spasticity of the quadriceps has been addressed by Gage et al., who recommended a medial transfer of the distal part of the rectus femoris to reduce the spasticity of the quadriceps after fractional hamstring lengthening [77]. The rectus femoris tendon is transferred medially to sartorius or semitendinosus or semimembranosus. The effect on rotation, however, is

minimal, and hence a lateral transfer is not recommended. This procedure increases the dynamic range of motion at the knee by about 15–20° [78] and is recommended in conjunction with fractional hamstring lengthening provided that co-spasticity of the hamstrings and rectus has been demonstrated. Knee hyperextension may result from previous surgery if the knee flexors become too weak. The hamstrings also control the position of the pelvis and excessive weakening may result in an increased anterior pelvic tilt and a compensatory lumbar hyperlordosis. If the knee hyperextension is due to spastic quadriceps, one solution is to perform a distal rectus tenotomy. Persisting crouch gait associated with patella alta, elongation of the patellar tendon, short hamstrings, and a knee capsular contracture can be managed by a supracondylar femoral extension osteotomy, patellar tendon shortening (or distal transfer of the tibial tuberosity if the tibial apophysis has closed), and fractional hamstring lengthening.

Foot and Ankle

These are common deformities. Equinus may be primarily caused by a contracture of the gastrocnemius or the soleus or be secondary to hip or knee flexion contractures. Whereas compensation for a knee flexion contracture requires hip flexion and vice versa, the position of the ankle is independent of the position of the hip and knee, provided the entire foot can make contact with the ground, either directly or indirectly via shoewear or a splint. Normal individuals can wear shoes of varying heel height and still maintain normal alignment of the hip and knee. Because hip and knee flexion results in a functional shortening of the leg, a compensatory equinus position is often used to allow foot contact. Therefore, the ankle should not be examined in isolation. The aim of treatment of an equinus deformity is to obtain full contact between the plantar aspect of the shoe and the ground and ensures that the shank is perpendicular to the floor in the standing position. Thus equinus can be accepted but requires a heel raise for compensation. In this situation additional stabilization by shoewear or an orthosis may be necessary. An AFO is especially helpful to compensate for drop foot deformity, as this is difficult to improve surgically.

If the equinus deformity is too severe or conservative treatment is not acceptable, the aim of management is to produce a plantigrade foot. Mild contracture of the calf muscles may respond to serial casting. Resting AFOs are widely used at night, but if tension is applied to improve dorsiflexion, there is usually poor compliance. Serial casting requires diligence and skill and may postpone the need for surgery. Applied injudiciously, serious damage can result

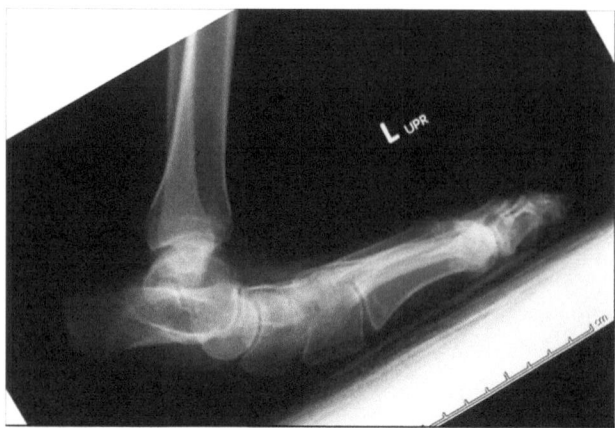

Fig. 6.12 Mid-foot break

if the foot is used as a lever to dorsiflex the ankle, producing a pseudo-correction at the expense of a mid-tarsal or hindfoot break (Fig. 6.12). To apply true stretch to the triceps surae muscle the subtalar joint must be locked by adduction–inversion in cases of valgus–abduction feet or the opposite in varus–adduction feet. If surgical lengthening of the triceps surae (Achilles tendon lengthening in hemiplegia or aponeurotic or gastrocnemius tendon lengthening or tenotomy in diplegia) is performed at an early age there is a likelihood of repeat surgery before skeletal maturity. Botulinum toxin injections can be used to lower tone and delay surgery. This has to be balanced against the disadvantages and social inconvenience of multiple visits for serial casting. Secondary deformities in the proximal lower limb, and the risk of iatrogenic overlengthening of the triceps muscle, are recognized risks. Flexible AFOs worn during function can maintain or even slightly improve dorsiflexion if plantar flexion is blocked and dorsiflexion is left free. These orthoses are superior to walking barefoot or with stiff orthoses [21].

In the assessment of equinus it is essential to distinguish, if possible, between tonic and phasic spasticity because the former is more capable of producing fixed contracture. Most operations are designed for muscle shortening resulting from tonic spasticity. Calf muscle force should be preserved as much as possible as the triceps surae controls standing posture, and its force is necessary for running, jumping, and stair climbing. Weakening this muscle might improve gait and heel posture relative to the floor but interferes with many other functions. Most centers now are cautious about lengthening the soleus in diplegia for fear of defunctioning the triceps. It is now considered safer to lengthen the gastrocnemius only in diplegia and to accept, if necessary, some residual equinus from a short soleus which can be compensated for by shoewear or a small heel raise. The gastrocnemius tendon can be divided using the Vulpius [79] or

Strayer [80] technique. In hemiplegia, however, there is often coexisting shortening of the gastrocnemius and soleus and so Achilles tendon lengthening here is permissible. Although the muscle itself is short, most surgeons perform an elongation of the tendo-Achilles and this may be done open or closed. A percutaneous Hoke technique is effective assuming that this is a primary procedure and that no other lengthenings in that region are required. Care must be taken, however, to prevent overlengthening as control of heel cord length may be difficult with this procedure. If a concomitant intramuscular tibialis posterior lengthening is required, the Achilles tendon procedure can be done by an open technique using a Z-lengthening. Repeated Achilles tendon lengthening can also be done percutaneously, providing the skin is not adherent to the underlying tendon. The tendon is tenotomized at three sites: one-half medially and distally, one-half medially and proximally, and one-half laterally between the two medial cuts. The tendon slides apart as the foot is dorsiflexed to no more than a right angle when holding the hindfoot in varus. A below-knee cast is then applied while the foot is held at a right angle, but not beyond, to avoid producing calcaneus. If less correction is required, aponeurotic lengthening, the Baumann procedure [81], is sufficient: the aponeuroses of the gastrocnemii and, if necessary, of the soleus are exposed in the middle third of the shank and are divided at three or four sites perpendicular to the fiber direction. This procedure does not produce a direct gain in muscle length, and hence post-operative physiotherapy is mandatory. The advantage of this procedure is the preservation of muscle strength [21, 22].

There are three common causes for pes varus: spasticity of the tibialis posterior, tibialis anterior, or of the gastrocnemius–soleus, or a combination of these. Gastrocnemius–soleus causes inversion of the ankle, whereas the tibialis posterior causes hindfoot varus, and tibialis anterior mid-foot varus. Indications for surgery in this group are failure of an orthosis to control the foot deformity, which is especially difficult if the deformity is produced during swing. Subsequent bony changes need to be prevented. A variety of procedures has been advocated. If there is no fixed joint deformity, the aim should be to balance the foot by procedures on the deforming musculotendinous units. Inversion at the ankle is corrected by judicious elongation of the tendo-Achilles in hemiplegia and of the gastrocnemius in diplegia. Inversion of the hindfoot can be corrected by either an intramuscular tibialis posterior lengthening [82] or a split tibialis posterior transfer [83]. The former can be accomplished through the same incision used for Achilles tendon or gastrocnemius surgery, which usually has to be performed as well. Simple tibialis posterior tenotomy is contraindicated for fear of producing a flat foot and valgus deformity. Inversion of the mid-foot is corrected by a split tibialis anterior tendon transfer [84, 85]. Alternatively, the whole tendon can be transferred to the dorsum or lateral side of the foot depending upon the correction required. The object is to balance muscle action across the medial and lateral sides of the foot. Fixed bony deformity requires a combination of soft tissue surgery and bony correction. For a fixed varus hind-foot a lateral closing wedge osteotomy of the calcaneus in addition to soft tissue surgery is indicated. For a fixed hind- and mid-foot a triple fusion may be indicated after soft tissue release, but it should be noted that patients with stiff feet can have difficulty walking on uneven ground. Pes valgus may be due to spasticity of the peroneal muscles or triceps surae, but a major factor is pathological torsional moments during gait. Unless treated, the deformity will progress from flexible to rigid and produce secondary hallux valgus. The foot deformity can be managed either conservatively by an AFO or surgically. The procedure of choice is a calcaneal lengthening (Evans procedure) which is effective as long as the foot is flexible. An alternative is the extra-articular subtalar fusion, and the Dennyson and Fulford modification of the Grice–Green technique [86] has proved very reliable. Should hallux valgus occur, this may be treated by a metatarsal osteotomy or metatarso-phalangeal fusion. The foot should not be considered in isolation and it is essential to check that the underlying cause for a foot or toe deformity does not lie more proximally.

In older children a flexion deformity of the great toe can be troublesome, producing pressure sores on the metatarso-phalangeal joint (MTPJ), interphalangeal joint (IPJ), or on the pulp of the toe. This deformity is best managed by Z-lengthening of the muscle causing the deformity, and in severe cases by fusion of the IPJ or MTPJ depending on the site of the deformity.

Upper Limb Surgery

Conservative Management

Indications for orthotic provision in the upper limb are rare. There are, however, two groups of patients who benefit from orthoses. In the first, spasticity of the muscles controlling wrist posture may position the hand out of the patient's direct field of vision which makes use of the hand difficult and in some patients finger and thumb function can be improved by stabilizing the wrist with a splint. In the second, patients present with progressive flexion deformity of the fingers and wrist, which interferes with care and nursing. These muscles often respond to stretching by a positional splint worn during the day. The splint needs to be adjusted regularly to maintain any gain in range of motion. Splinting for elbow and shoulder is difficult and cumbersome, and the rare successes hardly justify its use.

Surgery

Some patients, especially when older, develop severe flexion deformities in the upper limb at the wrist, elbow, and sometimes the shoulder. These contracted muscles can respond to injections of botulinum toxin A combined with stretching and positional orthoses.

Only a small number of patients are suitable for upper limb surgery. Assessment should be considered with the overall disability of the child and realistic goals set. Surgical procedures usually consist of positioning the arm in a more functional or cosmetic position. Important criteria for intervention include the intelligence, motivation, motor function, sensibility, and age [87]. As with the lower limb, muscle weakness, fixed deformity, dynamic deformity, and contractures need to be assessed. Similarly, a distinction should be made between phasic and tonic spasticity. Rigidity may produce either flexor or extensor dystonia. There is no reciprocal inhibition associated with dystonia so both agonists and antagonists grow normally and tendon transfers in this situation can produce the opposite and equally disabling posture. Poor sensibility does not exclude surgery, but poor stereognosis, two-point discrimination greater than 15–20 mm, and an inability to position the hand in space when the eyes are closed are relative contraindications to procedures designed to improve fine coordination [87]. Athetosis may make tendon transfers unreliable.

Operations in the upper limb include joint stabilization, release of contractures, musculotendinous lengthening, and tendon transfer. The usual deformity in the shoulder is adduction and internal rotation. Where there is a fixed contracture, derotation humeral osteotomy can improve elbow and forearm positions. Painful subluxation due to untreated shoulder deformity is rare. Elbow flexion contractures can cause severe functional problems. Loss of 30° of extension may not require treatment on its own, but if loss of elbow extension prevents efficient use of crutches or if the patient, who is usually hemiplegic, dislikes the appearance, surgical release can be effective. An anterior elbow release (Z-lengthening of biceps tendon, fractional lengthening of brachialis, and release of the flexor–pronator origin) can improve the contracture but care should be taken to avoid a fixed extension deformity. For daily activities it is usually more important for the patient to have sufficient flexion at the elbow to be able to reach the head and mouth than to have full elbow extension.

The following deformities may occur distal to the elbow: pronation of the forearm, wrist and finger flexion, and thumb adduction or "thumb-in-palm." In the forearm, pronation can be dealt with by pronator teres tenotomy if this is an isolated problem or can be combined with a flexor–pronator release [88] if there is a severe flexion deformity of the wrist and fingers. This operation produces an unselective release of all the flexors and should be reserved for severe deformity with no prospect of useful hand function; otherwise selective flexor lengthenings and transfers should be considered.

Excessive wrist flexion is a common deformity and inhibits hand grasp. Zancolli et al. have provided guidelines on the surgical management of wrist and finger flexion deformities, summarized below [89]. Wrist flexion is often associated with ulnar deviation, and tendon transfers can improve extension. Where there is mild spasticity, a tenotomy of the flexor carpi ulnaris and musculo-aponeurotic release of the flexor origins are recommended. If the wrist extensors are weak the flexor carpi ulnaris is transferred to extensor carpi radialis brevis.

Musculo-aponeurotic release of the flexors may also be necessary and where finger extension is only possible with the wrist flexed beyond 50°, an additional pronator release is recommended. Severe flexion of the fingers and an inability to extend the fingers in full wrist flexion may be treated by multiple tendon lengthenings in the forearm. Transfer of flexor carpi ulnaris to extensor digitorum communis has the advantage over the Green and Banks [90] transfer to extensor carpi radialis brevis in that it may not result in extension contractures of the fingers. Wrist arthrodesis is indicated for cosmesis in the nonfunctional hand and is usually requested by hemiplegics, for degenerative changes at the wrist with associated pain, or where there is functional finger flexion and extension when the wrist is immobilized in neutral. One technique is to use a contoured one-third tubular plate for aligning the third metacarpal with the radius after the articular surfaces have been denuded. One pitfall of arthrodesis in a functional hand is in those patients who rely on crutches or a wheelchair for mobility. They may not be able to use crutches efficiently once the wrist has been fused in the "optimum" position because they are unable to transfer body weight to the palm of the hand. Adduction contracture of the thumb can be treated by myotomy of the adductor muscle in the palm. This is preferred to tenotomy as it releases the first metacarpal but does not allow hyperextension of the metacarpo-phalangeal joint [91]. The thumb-in-palm deformity is complex and often difficult to treat. The main deforming force is the flexor pollicis longus but there may also be spasticity of the adductor pollicis, flexor pollicis brevis, or abductor pollicis brevis. To confirm that the flexor pollicis longus is the principal deforming force, thumb flexion should decrease on wrist flexion and conversely wrist extension will exaggerate the deformity. Several procedures are necessary to deal with the deformity: release of adductor pollicis, flexor pollicis brevis, and abductor pollicis brevis; arthrodesis of the metacarpophalangeal joint if unstable; lengthening of flexor pollicis longus; and re-routing of extensor pollicis longus [53, 87, 92].

Post-Operative Management and Complications

Immediate post-operative management will depend upon the type of procedure performed. Bony and tendon surgery will require a period of immobilization to allow tissue healing and to lessen the effects of muscle spasm. In the lower limb, calf muscle or tendon surgery can be undertaken as a day case and immediate weight-bearing in a below-knee plaster cast begun within the limits of comfort. Isolated hamstring and rectus femoris surgery requires the use of either a long leg cast or a lightweight removable splint. If the hamstrings are particularly tight, the knee is not extended to its limit but left in a slightly flexed position. A new cast is applied with the knee extended under general anesthesia 2 weeks later, after wound healing. Excessive stretch of the flexed knee has been reported to produce persistent neural damage [93]. Alternatively, a positional orthosis with an extendible knee mechanism can be used. The advantage is that stretch can be applied while the patient is conscious and adjustments made as necessary. The splint needs to be fitted before surgery and is worn 23 out of 24 h per day until the desired extension has been achieved. A hip spica or equivalent orthosis may be used after hip relocation surgery in the nonwalker.

In the immediate post-operative period careful consideration should be given to the relief of pain and spasm and the maintenance of the desired position of the limb. In the lower limb post-operative epidural anesthesia is highly desirable as it addresses these two main immediate problems and can be maintained for several days. The child should be mobilized as soon as is practicable.

Rehabilitation after surgery is lengthy, time consuming, and involves both the therapist and parents or carers. Recovery after even a minor procedure can take many months because of the new demands made on the neuromuscular system. It may take over a year to achieve maximum benefit after multiple-level surgery in the lower limb and the patient, parents, therapist, and surgeon can be frustrated by the apparent lack of progress after such procedures.

It should not be forgotten that CP is an incurable condition, and careful preoperative assessment is essential to avoid exchanging one problem for an even worse one. Therefore goals must be realistic. The need for surgery may coincide with unfavorable events occurring in the natural history of the child's development, such as diminishing efficiency of walking, and an indifferent outcome does not necessarily result from surgery but may appear to. The present trend toward multiple-level surgery at one sitting is justifiable provided that excellent preoperative assessment is made but does increase the possibility of error.

There are several pitfalls in the surgical management of CP apart from complications common to any surgical procedure. The most serious penalties result from inadequate assessment, performing operations at the wrong level, and failing to allow for the action of muscles that cross two joints. An example of this type of error is an Achilles tendon lengthening for an equinus attitude that is caused by a hip flexion contracture. Overlengthening of musculotendinous units may produce an even worse deformity; examples include calcaneus after excessive Achilles tendon lengthening, an excessively broad-based gait or, even worse, an abduction contracture at the hip after excessive adductor surgery. In principle it is better to correct proximal deformities first and to reassess the influence of this distally. Incorrect assessment of bony deformity can give poor results; for example, significant uncovering of the femoral head is unlikely to be remedied by muscle releases alone, and if relocation is contemplated it should be done before the appearance of significant femoral head deformity. Equally, in considering torsional deformity, neither the femur nor the tibia should be viewed in isolation; correction of excessive femoral internal torsion by external derotation osteotomy in the presence of compensatory external tibial torsion will exaggerate the clinical appearances of an externally rotated lower limb. Unpredictable results follow surgery for rigidity or phasic spasticity and after soft tissue procedures in the presence of fixed bony deformity.

Assessment of the child with CP is challenging, and surgery can be effective but should be seen as only one aspect in the comprehensive management of the patient.

References

1. Ingram TT. Paediatric aspects of cerebral palsy. Edinburgh: Livingstone; 1964.
2. Brown JK, Minns RA. Mechanisms of deformity in children with cerebral palsy. Sem Orthop 1989; 4:236–255.
3. Ghasia F, Brunstrom J, Gordon M, Tychsen L. Frequency and severity of visual sensory and motor deficits in children with cerebral palsy: gross motor function classification scale. Invest Ophthalmol Vis Sci 2008; 49:572–580.
4. Sanger TD, Kukke SN. Abnormalities of tactile sensory function in children with dystonic and diplegic cerebral palsy. J Child Neurol 2007; 22:289–293.
5. Nelson KB, Ellenberg JH. Antecedents of cerebral palsy. New Eng J Med 1986; 315:81–86.
6. Bejar R, Wozniak P, Ailard M , et al. Antenatal origin of neurologic damage in newborn infants. Preterm infants. Am J Obstet Gynecol 1988; 159:357–363.
7. Padilla-Gomes NF, Enríquez G, Acosta-Rojas R, et al. Prevalence of neonatal ultrasound brain lesions in premature infants with and without intrauterine growth restriction. Acta Paediatr 2007; 96:1582–1587.
8. Zimmerman RA, Bilaniuk LT. Neuroimaging evaluation of cerebral palsy. Clin Perinatol 2006; 33:517–544.
9. Sherrington C. The integrative action of the nervous system. New Haven CT Yale University Press; 1947.
10. Ziv I, Blackburn N, Rang M, Korerska J. Muscle growth in normal and spastic mice. Dev Med Child Neurol 1984; 26:94–99.
11. Tardieu C, Lespargot A, Tabary C, Bret MD. For how long must the soleus muscle be stretched each day to prevent contracture? Dev Med Child Neurol 1988; 30:3–10.
12. Levitt S. Treatment of Cerebral Palsy and Motor Delay, 4th ed. Oxford: Blackwell; 2004.
13. Staheli LT. The prone hip extension test. Clin Orthop Rel Res 1977; 123:12–15.
14. Ruwe PA, Gage JR, Ozonoff MB, DeLuca PA. Clinical determination of femoral anteversion. J Bone Joint Surg Am 1992; 74A:820–830.
15. Staheli LT, Engel GM. Tibial torsion. A method of assessment and a survey of normal children. Clin Orthop Rel Res 1972; 86:183–186.
16. Hazlewood ME, Simmons AN, Johnson WT, et al. The footprint method to assess transmalleolar axis. Gait Posture 2007; 25:597–603.
17. Perry J, Antonelli D, Plur J, et al. Electromyography before and after surgery for hip deformity in children with cerebral palsy. J Bone Joint Surg Am 1976; 58A:201–208.
18. Perry J, Hoffer MM, Giovan P, et al. Gait analysis of the triceps surae in cerebral palsy. J Bone Joint Surg Am 1974; 56A:511–520.
19. Gage JR. Gait analysis in cerebral palsy. Clinics in developmental medicine, no. 121. Oxford: MacKeith Press; 1947.
20. Read HS, Hazlewood ME, Hillman SJ, et al. Edinburgh Visual Gait Score for use in cerebral palsy. J Pediatr Orthop 2003; 23:296–301.
21. Brunner, R. Die Auswirkungen der Aponeurosendurchtrennung auf den Muskel. Habilitation-Dissertation, University of Basel, Basel, Switzerland, 1998.
22. Jaspers RT, Brunner R, Pel JJ, Huijing PA. Acute effects of intramuscular aponeurotomy on rat gastrocnemius medialis: force transmission, muscle force and sarcomere length. J Biomech 1999; 32:71–79.
23. Tardieu G, Thuilleux G, Tardieu C, Huet, et al. Tour E. Long term effects of surgical elongation of the tendo calcaneus in the normal cat. Develop Med Child Neurol 1979; 21:83–94.
24. Damiano DL, Kelly LE, Vaughn CL. Effects of quadriceps femoris muscle strengthening on crouch gait in children with spastic diplegia. Phys Ther 1995; 75:658–667.
25. Hullin MG, Robb JE, Loudon IR. Ankle-foot orthosis function in low-level myelomeningocele. J Pediatr Orthop 1992; 12: 518–521.
26. Brunner R, Meier G, Ruepp T. Comparison of a stiff and a spring-type ankle-foot orthosis to improve gait in spastic hemiplegic children. J Pediatr Orthop 1998; 18:719–726.
27. Farmer SE, Woollam PJ, Patrick JH, et al. Dynamic orthoses in the management of joint contracture. J Bone Joint Surg 2005; 87B:291–295.
28. Terjesen T, Lange JE, Steen H. Treatment of scoliosis with spinal bracing in quadriplegic cerebral palsy. Dev Med Child Neurol 2000; 42:448–454.
29. Tsirikos AI, Chang W-N, Dabney KW, Miller F. Comparison of parents' and caregivers' satisfaction after spinal fusion in children with cerebral palsy. J Pediatr Orthop 2004; 24:54–58.
30. Peacock WJ, Arens LJ, Goldberg MJ. Cerebral palsy spasticity. Selective posterior rhizotomy. Paediatr Neurosci 1987; 13:61–66.
31. Oppenheim WL. Selective posterior rhizotomy for spastic cerebral palsy. Clin Orthop Rel Res 1990; 253:20–29.
32. Spiegel DA, Loder RT, Alley KA, et al. Spinal deformity following selective dorsal rhizotomy. J Pediatr Orthop 2004; 24:30–36.
33. Greene WB, Dietz FR, Goldberg MJ, et al. Rapid progression of hip subluxation in cerebral palsy after selective posterior rhizotomy. J Pediatr Orthop 1991; 11:494–497.

34. Steinbok P. Selective dorsal rhizotomy for spastic cerebral palsy: a review. Childs Nerv Syst 2007; 23:981–990.

35. Farmer JP, Sabbagh AJ. Selective dorsal rhizotomies in the treatment of spasticity related to cerebral palsy. Childs Nerv Syst 2007; 23:991–1002.

36. Buckon CE, Thomas SS, Piatt JH Jr, et al. Selective dorsal rhizotomy versus orthopedic surgery: a multidimensional assessment of outcome efficacy. Arch Phys Med Rehabil 2004; 85:457–465.

37. Krach LE, Kriel RL, Gilmartin RC, et al. GMFM 1 year after continuous intrathecal baclofen infusion. Pediatr Rehabil 2005; 8:207–213.

38. Hoving MA, van Raak EP, Spincemaille GH, et al. Dutch Study Group on Child Spasticity. Intrathecal baclofen in children with spastic cerebral palsy: a double-blind, randomized, placebo-controlled, dose-finding study. Dev Med Child Neurol 2007; 49:654–659.

39. Albright AL. Intrathecal baclofen for childhood hypertonia. Childs Nerv Syst 2007; 23:971–979.

40. Ginsburg GM, Lauder AJ. Progression of scoliosis in patients with spastic quadriplegia after the insertion of an intrathecal baclofen pump. Spine 2007; 32:2745–2750.

41. Senaran H, Shah SA, Presedo A, et al. The risk of progression of scoliosis in cerebral palsy patients after intrathecal baclofen therapy. Spine 2007; 32:2348–2354.

42. Cosgrove AP, Graham HK. Botulinum toxin A prevents the development of contractures in the hereditary spastic mouse. Dev Med Child Neurol 1994, 36:379–385.

43. Koman LA, Mooney JF 3rd, Smith BP, et al. Management of spasticity in cerebral palsy with botulinum-A toxin: report of a preliminary, randomized, double-blind trial. J Pediatr Orthop 1994, 14:299–303.

44. Molenaers G, Desloovere K, Fabry G, De Cock P. The effects of quantitative gait assessment and botulinum toxin a on musculoskeletal surgery in children with cerebral palsy. J Bone Joint Surg Am 2006; 88A:161–170.

45. James JIP. Paralytic scoliosis. J Bone Joint Surg Br 1956; 38B:660–685.

46. Lonstein JE, Beck K. Hip dislocation and subluxation in cerebral palsy. J Pediatr Orthop 1986; 6:521–526.

47. Madigan RR, Wallace SL. Scoliosis in cerebral palsy: short term follow-up and prognosis in untreated institutionalized patients. Orthop Trans 1986; 10:17.

48. Thomas KJ, Simon SR. Progression of scoliosis after skeletal maturity in institutionalized adults who have cerebral palsy. J Bone Joint Surg Am 1988; 70A:1290–1296.

49. Dabney KW, Miller F, Lipton GE, et al. Correction of sagittal plane spinal deformities with unit rod instrumentation in children with cerebral palsy. J Bone Joint Surg Am 2004; 86A:156–168.

50. Miller F. Spinal deformity secondary to impaired neurologic control. J Bone Joint Surg Am 2007; 89A:143–147.

51. Soo B, Howard JJ, Boyd RN, Reid SM, Lanigan A, Wolfe R, Reddihough D, Graham HK. Hip displacement in cerebral palsy. J Bone Joint Surg [Am] 2006; 88A:121–9.

52. Graham HK, Boyd RN, Carlin JB, et al. Does botulinum toxin A combined with bracing prevent hip displacement in children with cerebral palsy and 'hips at risk'? A randomized, controlled trial. J Bone Joint Surg Am 2008; 90A:23–33.

53. Bleck EE. Orthopaedic management in cerebral palsy. Clinics in Developmental Medicine, no. 99/100. London: Mac Keith Press; 1987.

54. Reimers J. The stability of the hip in children. A radiological study of the results of muscle surgery in spastic cerebral palsy. Acta Orthopaedica Scandinavica (Supplement) 1980; 184:1–97.

55. Faraj S, Atherton WG, Stott NS. Inter- and intra-measurer error in the measurement of Reimers' hip migration percentage. J Bone Joint Surg Br 2004; 86B:434–437.

56. Howard CB, Williams LA. A new radiological sign in the hips of cerebral palsy patients. Clin Radiol 1984; 35:317–319.

57. Heinrich SD, MacEwan GD, Zembo MM. Hip dysplasia, subluxation and dislocation in cerebral palsy: an arthrographic analysis. J Pediatr Orthop 1991; 11:488–493.

58. Brunner R, Picard C, Robb JE. Morphology of the acetabulum in hip dislocations due to cerebral palsy. J Pediatr Orthop Part B 1997; 6:207–211.

59. Brunner R, Baumann JU. Clinical benefit of reconstruction of dislocated and subluxated hip joints in patients with spastic cerebral palsy. J Pediatr Orthop 1994; 14:290–294.

60. Brunner R, Döderlein L. Pathological fractures in patients with cerebral palsy. J Pediatr Orthop Part B 1996; 5:232–238.

61. Cooperman DR, Bartucci E, Dierrick E, Millar EA. Hip dislocation in spastic cerebral palsy: long-term consequences. J Pediatr Orthop 1987; 7:268–276.

62. Noonan KJ, Jones J, Pierson J, et al. Hip function in adults with severe cerebral palsy. J Bone Joint Surg Am 2004; 86A:2607–2613.

63. Dobson F, Boyd RN, Parrott J, et al. Hip surveillance in children with cerebral palsy. Impact on the surgical management of spastic hip disease J Bone Joint Surg Br 2002; 84B:720–726.

64. Kalen V, Bleck EE. Prevention of spastic paralytic dislocation of the hip. Dev Med Child Neurol 1985; 27:17–24.

65. Schmale GA, Eilert RE, Chang F, Seidel K. High reoperation rates after early treatment of the subluxating hip in children with spastic cerebral palsy. J Pediatr Orthop 2006; 26:617–623.

66. Pemberton PA. Pericapsular osteotomy of the ilium for treatment of congenital subluxation and dislocation of the hip. J Bone Joint Surg Am 1965; 47A:65–86.

67. Mubarak SJ, Valencia FG, Wenger DR. One-stage correction of the spastic dislocated hip. Use of pericapsular acetabuloplasty to improve coverage. J Bone Joint Surg Am 1992; 74A:1347–1357.

68. Robb JE, Brunner R. A Dega-type osteotomy after closure of the triradiate cartilage in non-walking patients with severe cerebral palsy. J Bone Joint Surg Br 2006; 88B:933–937.

69. Hogan KA, Blake M, Gross RH. Subtrochanteric valgus osteotomy for chronically dislocated, painful spastic hips. J Bone Joint Surgery Am 2007; 88A:2624–2631.

70. Castle ME, Schneider C. Proximal femoral resection-interposition arthroplasty. J Bone Joint Surg Am 1978; 60A:1051–1054.

71. Rodda JM, Graham HK, Nattrass GR, et al. Correction of severe crouch gait in patients with spastic diplegic with use of multilevel orthopaedic surgery. J Bone Joint Surg Am 2006; 88A:2653–2664.

72. Schwartz MH, Viehweger E, Stour J, et al. Comprehensive treatment of ambulatory children with cerebral palsy. An outcome assessment. J Pediatr Orthop 2004; 24:45–53.

73. Cuomo AV, Gamradt SC, Kim CO, et al. Health-related quality of life outcomes improve after multilevel surgery in ambulatory children with cerebral palsy. J Pediatr Orthop 2007; 27:653–657.

74. Pirpiris M, Trivett A, Baker R, et al. Femoral derotation osteotomy in spastic diplegia: proximal or distal? J Bone Joint Surg Br 2003; 85B:265–272.

75. Fabry G. Torsion of the femur. Acta Orthop Belg 1977; 43:454–459.

76. Brunner R, Baumann JU. Long term effects of intertrochanteric varus-derotation osteotomy on femur and acetabulum in spastic cerebral palsy. J Pediatr Orthop 1997; 17:585–591.

77. Gage JR, Perry J, Hicks RR, et al. Rectus femoris transfer to improve knee function of children with cerebral palsy. Dev Med Child Neurol 1987; 29:159–166.

78. Abel MF, Damiano DL, Pannunzio M, Bush J. Muscle-tendon surgery in diplegic cerebral palsy: functional and mechanical changes. J Pediatr Orthop 1999; 19:366–375.

79. Vulpius O, Stoffel A. Tenotomie der Endsehnen der Mm. gastrocnemius et soleus. Orthopädische Operationslehre. Stuttgart: Verlag von Ferdinand Enke; 1913:29–31.

80. Strayer LM. Recession of the gastrocnemius. An operation to relieve spastic contracture of the calf muscles. J Bone Joint Surg Am 1950; 32A:671–676.

81. Baumann JU, Koch HG. Ventrale aponeurotische Verlängerung des Musculus gastrocnemius. Operative Orthop Traumatol 1989; 1:254–258.

82. Ruda R, Frost HM. Cerebral palsy spastic varus and forefoot adductus, treated by intramuscular posterior tibial lengthening. Clin Orthop Rel Res 1971; 79:61–70.

83. Green NE, Griffen PP, Shiavi P. Split posterior tibial tendon transfer in spastic cerebral palsy. J Bone Joint Surg Am 1983; 65A:748–754.

84. Hoffer MM, Barakat G, Koffman M. 10-year follow-up of split anterior tibial tendon transfer in cerebral palsied patients with spastic equino-varus deformity. J Pediatr Orthop 1985; 5: 432–434.

85. Barnes MJ, Herring JA. Combined split anterior tibial-tendon transfer and intramuscular lengthening of the posterior tibial tendon. J Bone Joint Surg 1991; 73A:734–738.

86. Dennyson WG, Fulford GE. Subtalar arthrodesis by cancellous grafts and metallic internal fixation. J Bone Joint Surg Br 1976; 58B:507–510

87. Koman AL, Gelberman RH, Toby EB, Poehling GG. Cerebral palsy: management of the upper extremity. Clin Orthop Rel Res 1990; 253:62–74.

88. Page CM. An operation for the relief of flexion-contracture in the forearm. J Bone Joint Surg 1923; 5:233–234.

89. Zancolli EA, Goldner JL, Swanson AB. Surgery of the spastic hand in cerebral palsy; report of the committee on spastic hand evaluation. J Hand Surg 1983; 8:766–772.

90. Green WT, Banks HH. Flexor carpi ulnaris transplant and its use in cerebral palsy. J Bone Joint Surg Am 1962; 44A:1343–1352.

91. Matev I. Surgical treatment of spastic 'thumb-in-palm' deformity. J Bone Joint Surg Br 1963; 45B:703–708.

92. Goldner JL, Koman AL, Gelberman R, et al. Arthrodesis of the metacarpophalangeal joint in children and adults. Adjunctive treatment of thumb in palm deformity in cerebral palsy. Clin Orthop Rel Res 1990; 253:75–89.

93. Aspen RM, Porter RW. Nerve traction during correction of knee flexion deformity. A case report and calculation. J Bone Joint Surg Br 1994; 76-B:471–473.

Chapter 7

Arthrogryposis multiplex congenita

John A. Fixsen

Introduction

Arthrogryposis multiplex congenita literally means multiple curved joints, occurring as a congenital anomaly in the newborn. The first description is ascribed to Otto in 1841 [1]. Sheldon in 1932 published the first detailed description in the United Kingdom and called the condition "amyoplasia congenita" emphasizing the lack of muscle development in this condition [2]. It is important to realize that arthrogryposis is a descriptive term and not an exact diagnosis. Hall who has made a special study of the genetics of the disorder pointed out that there are at least 150 possible diagnoses that can result in multiple curved joint deformities in the newborn child [3]. The reader is referred to Hall for a comprehensive discussion of the disorder [4].

The features of the condition are multiple rigid joint deformities with defective muscles but normal sensation (Fig. 7.1). In the classical form, called amyoplasia congenita by Sheldon, all four limbs are involved, but the condition can also occur only in the upper limbs or only in the lower limbs. Hall et al. described a distal form in which the hands and feet are severely deformed with only minor contractures more proximally, although the spine may develop scoliosis [5]. This form is important, as it can be inherited as an autosomal dominant, whereas the majority of forms of classic arthrogryposis do not have a genetic background. At birth, the children can look terribly deformed and the parents are often horrified by the appearance of their child. In addition to the multiple rigid joint contractures, the skin lacks creases and deep dimples over the joints are very characteristic (Fig. 7.2). The limbs are tubular and featureless, but the trunk may be affected, giving a characteristic "wooden doll" appearance. Other congenital anomalies such as cryptorchidism, hernias, gastroschisis, and bowel atresia may also occur.

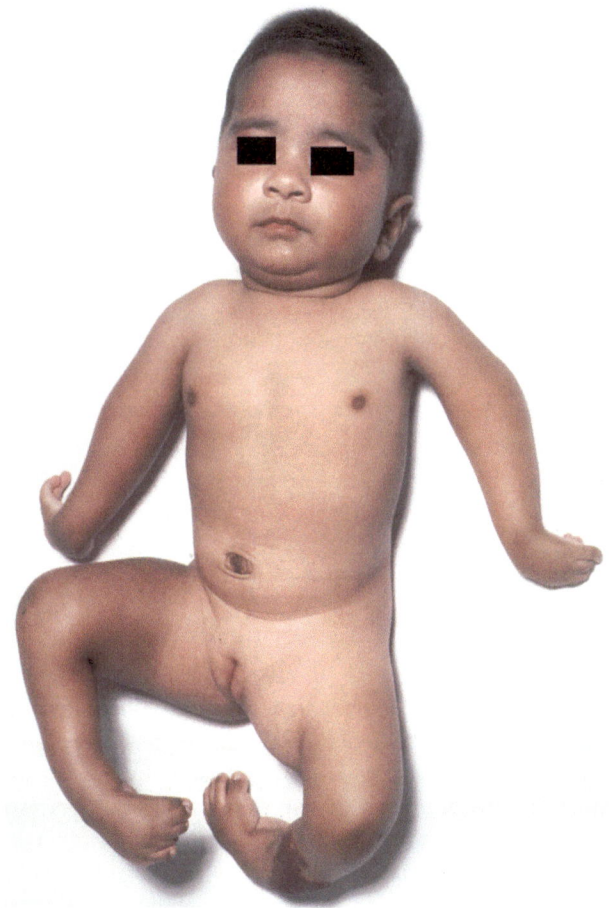

Fig. 7.1 Typical appearance of a child with four-limb arthrogryposis. Note adduction and internal rotation at the shoulders, extension at the elbows and flexion of the wrists, fixed flexion of the knees, and severe equinovarus feet

J.A. Fixsen (✉)
Orthopaedic Department, Great Ormond Street Hospital for Sick Children, London, UK

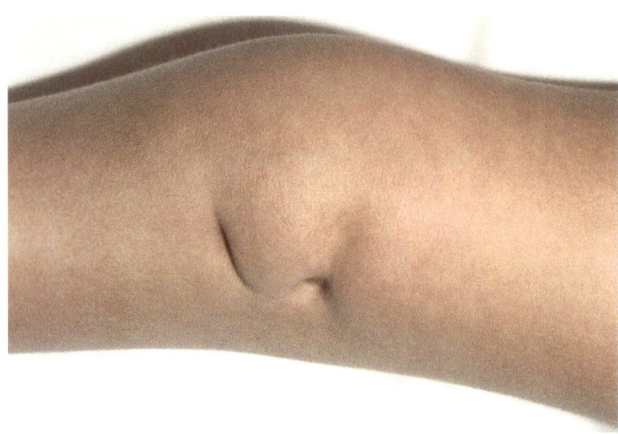

Fig. 7.2 Clinical photograph of the knee showing typical deep skin dimples

Incidence

The reported incidence varies widely, probably because arthrogryposis is a descriptive term that may be applied to all patients with stiff curved joints or only to those in whom there is no ascertainable cause after careful investigation. In Helsinki, an incidence of 3 per 10,000 live births was reported, but in the Edinburgh birth register, there was only 1 case in 56,000 live births. Wynne-Davies et al. looked at the incidence in the United Kingdom, Australia, and the United States and showed there was an apparent increase in the 1960 s, which suggested an infective cause for this unusual condition [6]. Hall quotes an incidence of classical arthrogryposis multiplex congenita (amyoplasia congenita) of 1 in 10,000 live births [4].

Etiology

There are many causes of arthrogryposis. Animal studies have shown that limitation of intrauterine movement can lead to a contracture at birth. Intrauterine infection by the Akabane virus in sheep, cows, and horses can produce a condition very similar to classical arthrogryposis. Mothers of babies born with multiple contractures often note decreased intrauterine mobility of the fetus. The factors that predispose to decreased intrauterine mobility include neuromuscular and connective tissue disorders, fetal crowding, oligohydramnios, multiple pregnancy, and malposition such as breech presentation.

An interesting case is reported of a pregnant mother treatment with curare for severe tetanus who gave birth to an arthrogrypotic baby. Wynne-Davies et al. concluded that the best description of the etiology was "an environmental disease of early pregnancy associated with one or more unfavorable intrauterine factors" [6].

Diagnosis

The paediatrician or orthopaedic surgeon presented with a child with arthrogrypotic features must first try to establish the diagnosis. The parents of the child are, not surprisingly, often extremely upset by the appearance of their child and want immediate answers to the cause of their child's deformity. However, parental counseling should be approached with care, particularly with regard to prognosis and possible treatment, until the etiology has been elucidated. It is not uncommon for anxious parents to be given an extremely pessimistic prognosis before the diagnosis is fully understood. Conversely, an overoptimistic prognosis can also be misleading if the child subsequently proves to have a severe underlying cause for the arthrogrypotic deformities.

The following investigations should be considered:

- Radiographs of the whole spine and computed tomography (CT) of the head
- Chromosome analysis
- Collagen biochemistry
- Plasma creatine kinase estimation to exclude myopathic disorders
- Electromyography (EMG) and nerve conduction studies
- Muscle and nerve biopsy

Possible *differential diagnoses* can be considered under the following headings.

Neurological Disorders

1. Spina bifida and spinal dysraphism in all its forms
2. Myelodysplasia
3. Sacral and lumbar agenesis (Fig. 7.3)
4. Spinal muscular atrophy
5. Fetal neuropathy

Muscle Disorders

1. Dystrophia myotonica
2. Congenital muscular dystrophy
3. Fetal myopathy
4. Fetal myasthenia

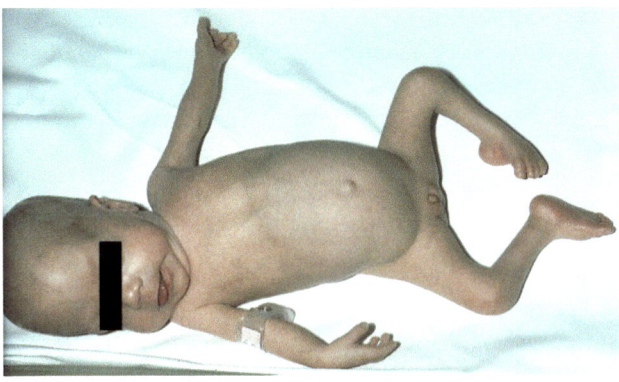

Fig. 7.3 Infant with sacral agenesis. Note how similar the lower limbs are to those in the arthrogrypotic child in Fig. 7.1

Connective Tissue Disorders

1. Marfan's syndrome
2. Ehlers–Danlos syndrome

Miscellaneous Syndromes

1. Freeman–Sheldon syndrome (cranio-carpo-tarsal dystrophy)
2. Turner's syndrome
3. Edward's syndrome (trisomy 18)
4. The pterygium or popliteal web syndrome
5. Diastrophic dwarfism

Bevan et al. suggests a multi-disciplinary team including a geneticist, paediatric orthopaedic surgeon, paediatric physiotherapist, and paediatric occupational therapist is very important both in establishing the diagnosis and the subsequent successful management of the child [7].

In general, classic amyoplasia congenita is not inherited, except for the distal form [5] affecting the hands and feet, which is commonly inherited as an autosomal dominant.

Orthopaedic Management

From the orthopaedic point of view, it is important to see these patients as soon as possible. Although it will take some time to establish the exact diagnosis, it is important to start treating the deformities early, as some of them will respond remarkably well to physiotherapy, stretching, and splintage. Some of the patients may be born with fractures and need treatment. However intractable a deformity may appear, it

is worth trying gentle manipulation and simple splintage, much of which can be done by the parents under the supervision of the physiotherapist in the first few months of life [8]. This strategy can also be very helpful in coping with the understandable parental concern. The parents must be told, however, that simple conservative treatment with stretching and splintage is unlikely to correct the deformities completely. Significant gains are especially likely in the hands, and often the knees and elbows.

In general, the limb deformities tend to be more severe distally. The feet and hands are nearly always involved, but the hips and shoulders may be quite mobile. None the less, if the hips are involved this is often with irreducible dislocation. The application of early splintage to such hips should be avoided, as it may cause avascular necrosis and increase the child's disability. Many of these children are rather weak and floppy in the first few months of life. Robinson has pointed out that they have significant problems with feeding, swallowing, sucking, weight gain, and recurrent chest infections in the first year of life [9]. Corrective surgery should be delayed until it is clear that the child is thriving and is developing trunk and sitting balance.

If orthopaedic deformities are corrected early, they must be rigorously splinted. There is a very strong tendency for recurrent deformity unless the corrected position can be adequately held by splintage. This can be very difficult in the small, tubular, featureless limbs that characterize this condition. Lower limb deformities that inhibit or prevent standing and walking by the time the child shows evidence of wanting to do so should be corrected if possible by the age of 18 months to 2 years.

In the upper limb, a careful assessment of overall function should be made before any decision regarding surgery. This usually means waiting until the age of 4 or 5 years, and a considerable period of observation and assessment. The use of special tools and utensils, assessment, and education by an experienced paediatric occupational therapist are often preferable to a complex operation, which may improve one joint but introduce other problems for the child because of the overall nature of the disorder [10, 11].

Orthopaedic Management of the Lower Limbs

The Foot

The foot is usually in fixed severe equinovarus (Fig. 7.1). Less commonly, a congenital vertical talus deformity is present. Serial stretching and strapping or splintage using the Ponseti method (see Chapter 31) may sometimes correct the deformity. However, frequently the foot is completely incorrigible and shows no response to conservative treatment. Once it is clear that conservative treatment will not be successful, surgery should be considered, preferably when the child is ready to walk. The foot is likely to require an extensive soft tissue release involving the medial, posterior, and lateral structures, which is best performed through the Cincinnati approach. If the foot fails to correct fully with even the most extensive soft tissue release or relapses quickly within 2–3 years, talectomy may have to be considered.

Talectomy has produced good results in these stiff, rigid feet [12–14]. The talus is best approached through a lateral incision, as for a triple arthrodesis. The important details are as follows. First, the entire talus must be removed. This can be difficult, because the normal tissue planes are poorly developed and the anatomy distorted, particularly if previous extensive soft tissue surgery has been performed. Second, it is important to find the ankle joint early during the operation and work round the talus, avoiding cutting into the talus itself or the tibia and malleoli. The posterior structures form an inextensile tether, and it is sensible not simply to lengthen the tendo-Achilles but to excise a 1-cm length of the fibrous cord that represents the tendo-Achilles posteriorly. Once the talus has been removed, the os calcis should be stabilized below the tibia by a K-wire, driven up through the heel pad and calcaneus into the tibia and retained for 6 weeks. Talectomy produces a plantigrade foot that is inevitably stiff and requires long-term splintage.

Recurrent deformity after talectomy is difficult to treat. The flexor hallucis longus is often tight, and it should be divided distally at the level of the metatarso-phalangeal joint of the big toe to prevent troublesome flexion of the toe. Talectomy cannot influence forefoot adduction, and if this persists and is symptomatic, a lateral calcaneocuboid fusion can be considered. Spontaneous fusion of the calcaneus to the tibia occurs in some patients but does not cause problems provided the calcaneus is in a satisfactory neutral position.

The Ilizarov technique and apparatus offer the opportunity of correcting complex foot deformities in three dimensions. Grill and Franke [15] reported the use of the Ilizarov apparatus in nine severely deformed feet, with satisfactory results in terms of function and appearance; one of their patients suffered from arthrogryposis [9]. More recently Reinke and Carpenter reported that Ilizarov application in the paediatric foot achieved satisfactory results in 21 of 24 feet; three of their patients suffered from arthrogryposis [16].

The rarer congenital vertical talus (see Chapter 33) is approached through a Cincinnati incision, allowing a posterior release, reduction of the talo-navicular dislocation, and lengthening of the tight lateral structures. The corrected position is held with K-wires. This operation produces a satisfactory stiff plantigrade foot for walking. Again, there is no urgency to rush into operation because the child can stand

very well on a rocker-bottomed foot and, if necessary, the operation can be deferred until other procedures on the hip and knee have been carried out.

The Knee

The knee presents with one of two problems: either severe fixed flexion (Fig. 7.1) or fixed extension (Fig. 7.4). Both deformities should be treated initially by repeated stretching and splintage, supervised by the physiotherapist. Surprisingly good results can be obtained in apparently rigid deformities. If the deformity does not respond to soft tissue stretching, surgery must be considered [17]. It is most important to plan surgery for the knee in relation to treatment of the foot. If the foot requires immobilization with the knee flexed, then attempts to straighten a flexed knee should wait until the foot has been treated. Conversely, if the knee is in fixed extension, it is often better to correct the knee

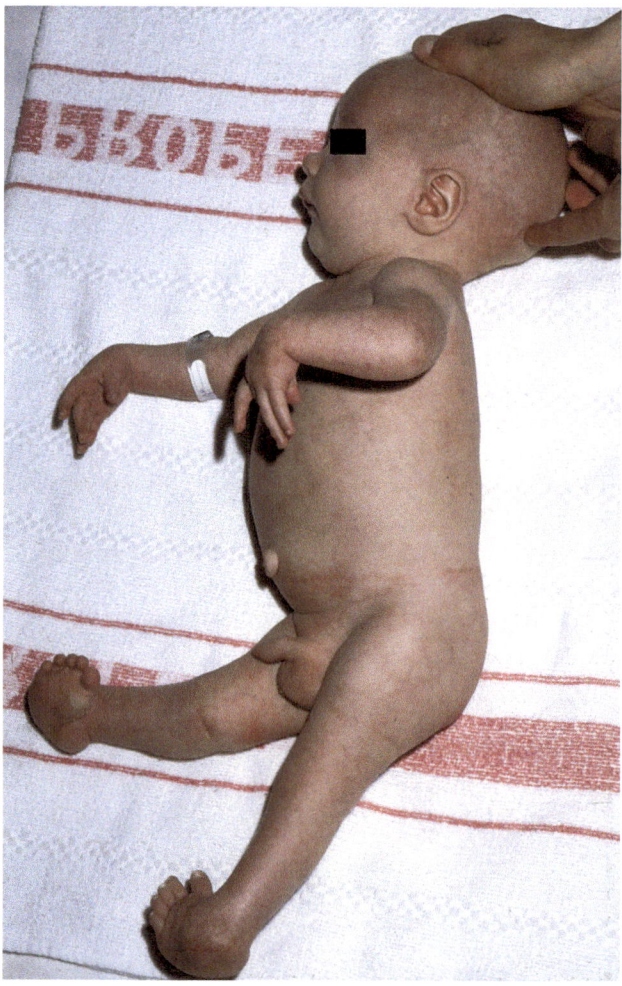

Fig. 7.4 Infant with arthrogryposis and fixed extended knees

extension before operation on the foot, so that the foot can be immobilized with a flexed knee.

In general, most joints in arthrogryposis have a relatively fixed arc of movement, and the aim of surgery is to transfer that arc into the most useful range rather than hoping to gain a significant improvement. Although occasionally there is a very gratifying improvement in the overall range, the main aim of treatment is to convert, for instance, a range of movement at the knee from fixed flexion of 90° with further flexion to 130°, to a range of flexion from 5 to 45°— a much more useful range for walking and acceptable for sitting. The operation for fixed flexion involves an extensive posterior release of all the soft tissue structures except the neurovascular bundle at the back of the knee. Usually it is not possible to use a tourniquet because of the small size of the child's leg. It is essential to divide all the structures that are tight. Medial and lateral incisions, rather than a midline longitudinal incision, should be used to minimize problems with wound healing when the knee is extended. The heads of the gastrocnemii and the posterior capsule of the knee joint are usually a significant part of the contracture and should be divided. Sometimes the posterior cruciate has to be released. Instability is rarely a problem because these joints are inherently stiff and the patient will have to wear an orthosis for many years to maintain correction. It is often impossible to extend the knee fully immediately because of the tightness of the neurovascular bundle; serial plasters over a period of weeks can slowly improve the range of extension. Once this is gained, splintage for many years is necessary to maintain knee extension (Fig. 7.5). Sometimes, in older children who have not had early soft tissue surgery, it is not possible to extend the knee without jeopardizing the blood supply to the lower leg. In this situation an extension and shortening osteotomy of the distal femur to produce relative lengthening of the soft tissues can be used to obtain full extension at the knee. Occasionally if there is gross bony deformity at the knee, fusion to correct the deformity may be considered. It is extremely tempting to consider supracondylar osteotomy to obtain correction and to ease the problem of the soft tissues. Unfortunately unless this is delayed until near maturity, the patient may develop, with growth, an extremely ugly and awkward angular deformity at the site of the osteotomy (Fig. 7.6). In general, osteotomies for the correction of deformity in arthrogryposis should be delayed until near maturity to avoid progressive or recurrent deformity.

Fixed hyperextension of the knee may respond remarkably well to serial stretching and splintage [17]. If there is no response to conservative treatment, a quadricepsplasty comprising an extensive dissection of the scarred and fibrotic quadriceps muscle is necessary to obtain some flexion at the knee. Long-term splintage is likely to be necessary to protect and support the knee after this type of surgery unless

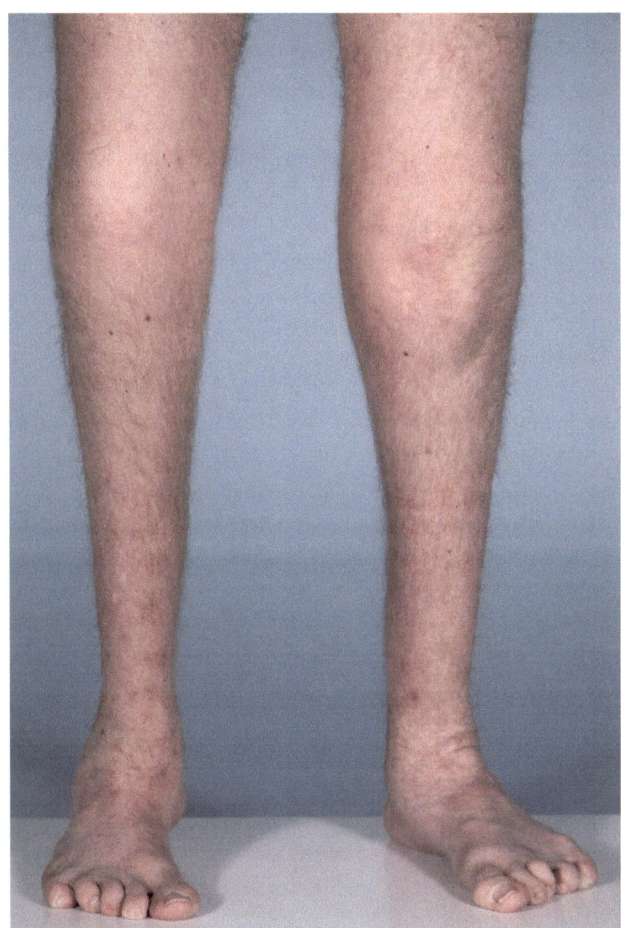

Fig. 7.5 Child after treatment for fixed flexion of the knees and several years splintage.

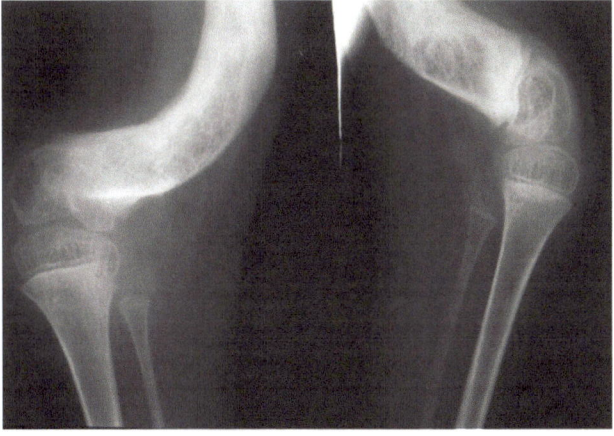

Fig. 7.6 Lateral radiographs of both knees showing severe posterior angulation of the femur above the knee following supracondylar osteotomies several years earlier

there is at least quadriceps power of grade 3 or more [18]. For this reason Parsch and Pietrzak prefer not to lengthen the quadriceps if the muscle is too weak to stabilize the knee post-operatively without braces [19].

The Ilizarov apparatus would appear to be an attractive alternative to difficult surgery with a high recurrence rate in the knee. However, Damsin and Trousseau [20] and Brunner et al. [21] point out the difficulties and high recurrence rate, particularly in young children, with this method. Nevertheless, it provides a useful alternative to surgery after failed physiotherapy, particularly in the older patient or the patient in whom previous surgery has failed.

The Hip

Frequently, one or both hips are dislocated. The clinical diagnosis can be very difficult. The general stiffness of the joints may make it impossible to perform the clinical tests for hip instability. There is often marked limitation of abduction, and a radiograph or ultrasound of the hips is necessary to decide whether they are displaced. If the hips are dislocated, they are rarely reducible on abduction and should not be splinted if irreducible. Splinting an unreduced hip is liable to cause avascular necrosis. If one hip is reduced and the other dislocated, it is worth surgically reducing the dislocated hip. If both hips are dislocated, Lloyd-Roberts and Lettin advised that they should be left alone, as it was rarely possible to get a satisfactory result on both sides, and the complication rate, particularly stiffness and recurrent dislocation, was high [22]. In 1987, Staheli et al. reported a small series of patients in whom reduction through the medial approach was performed in 25 hips, 7 of which were unilateral and 9 bilateral [23]. The majority of these operations were undertaken in children younger than 1 year. In a 5–6 year follow-up of these patients Szoke et al. reported only one redislocation and two cases of increased stiffness [24]. In contrast, Akazawa et al. recommended an extensive anterolateral approach to the hip and reported satisfactory results in a small series of patients followed for a mean of 11.8 years [25]. In the author's small experience of the medial approach, when successful, this does not appear to cause increased stiffness, but redislocation can occur, particularly if the hip is very dysplastic. Experience of extensive open reduction with femoral shortening has not always produced a stable, mobile hip. Yau et al. reported a 20-year follow-up of hip problems in arthrogryposis showing that open reduction was successful in stabilizing the hip but the hips were usually stiffer [26]. Adult patients with arthrogryposis and bilateral stable but completely dislocated hips tend to manage very well. If surgery is undertaken for bilateral dislocation and is not successful on both sides the result for the patient is often worse than if the hips had been left untreated

Apart from dislocation, the hips may be fixed in a very awkward frog or "Buddha" position of abduction and external rotation (Fig. 7.7). Fortunately, the conservative measures for the deformities in the lower limb distal to the

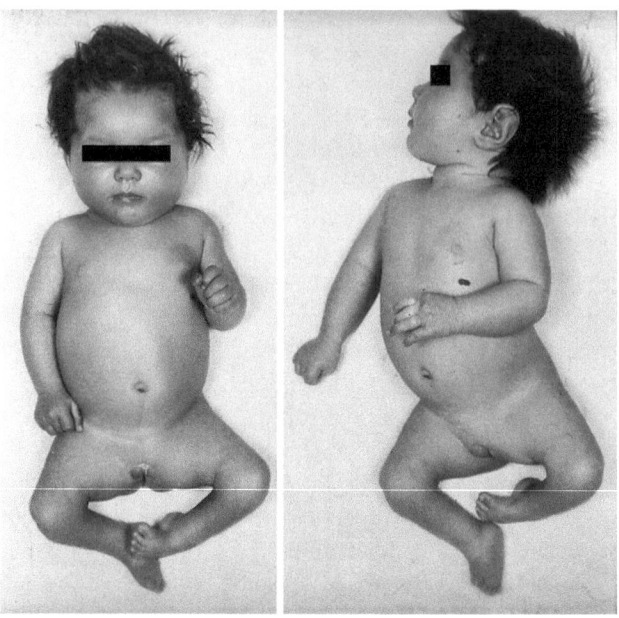

Fig. 7.7 Child showing the flexed abducted hips and flexed knees of the so-called Buddha position

hip, such as the plasters and splintage necessary for treating the feet and knees, help to stretch the hips, making it usually unnecessary to perform soft tissue release or corrective osteotomies to bring the hips into a neutral position. Fixed flexion of the hips is very common. It may require release, but when combined with some flexion at the knee it is often best left alone. As always in arthrogryposis, it is important to consider the treatment of the whole limb and not a single joint in isolation.

Orthopaedic Management of the Upper Limbs

As stated in the introduction, because of the complex interactions of all the deformities in the upper limb and the child's ability to develop remarkable trick movements, surgery should be considered very carefully and probably delayed at least until the child is aged about 4 years [27]. Physiotherapy has a major role in obtaining as much movement as possible at all the joints, especially in the fingers and wrists, where stretching and night splintage in the first year of life can be very helpful. Careful assessment by a skilled physiotherapist or occupational therapist should always be undertaken before making decisions about surgery.

The Shoulder

Weakness around the shoulder is very common. The characteristic position is adduction and internal rotation (Fig. 7.1).

Surgical intervention is rarely indicated although a simple external rotation osteotomy of the upper humerus will bring the hand and forearm into a more useful functional position.

The Elbow

At the elbow, the two common positions are fixed extension with little or no flexion (Fig. 7.8) and fixed flexion with little or no extension. Both deformities respond quite well to physiotherapy, but surgery may have to be considered once the child is established in walking. Activities such as using crutches and reaching the perineum for toileting require active extension of the elbow. The same applies to the ability to push oneself out of a chair, and so it is very important not to jeopardize active extension in the elbows by surgery designed to improve active flexion. If it is clear, once the child is walking, that it would be valuable to increase flexion in the elbow, there are three methods of gaining active flexion once passive flexion has been achieved.

Passive flexion is achieved by a posterior release of the elbow, lengthening the triceps, and releasing the posterior capsule and the collateral ligaments. This can be a very rewarding procedure and produces a useful arc of movement that allows the child to get hand to mouth without losing too much extension. Many children find that they can use passive flexion extremely well and do not particularly want to have an operation to provide active flexion if it means that they will lose active extension.

Once a reasonable range of passive flexion has been established, active motor power can be provided in the following ways:

1. If the forearm flexors and extensors are sufficiently strong, a Steindler flexorplasty advancing the flexor origin up the

humerus, and reinforcing this if necessary by advancing the extensor origin, is satisfactory. The problem with this operation is that, often, the muscles are not sufficiently strong to give useful flexion, and it may adversely affect the function of the fingers and wrist.

2. Triceps transfer was initially popularized by Williams [10]. In this operation, the triceps tendon is transferred to the radius and is a very strong active flexor. However, there is loss of active extension, which could be devastating for those patients requiring crutches or to push out of a wheelchair. Another troublesome complication is increasing fixed flexion, which may develop with time after this transfer, so that it is now rarely, if ever, used.

3. Pectoralis major transfer into the biceps tendon can be used but unfortunately the reported results deteriorate with progressive flexion deformity as the child grows [28]. If the biceps tendon is not present a modified Clark type of transfer will be necessary [22]. This requires mobilizing the pectoralis major low down on the chest wall and produces an extensive and unsightly scar.

The Wrist and Hand

The wrist is frequently fixed in flexion and the fingers curved and relatively immobile (Fig. 7.9). Manipulation and splintage in the first year of life can produce remarkable improvement in the range of movement. The thumb is often adducted and should be stretched out of the palm. Operations to correct wrist deformity have been described, such as partial or complete carpectomy or a dorsal wedge carpectomy. However, with growth, recurrence is very common. Fortunately, the flexed position of the wrist is very functional in these children, and often an advantage rather than a disadvantage.

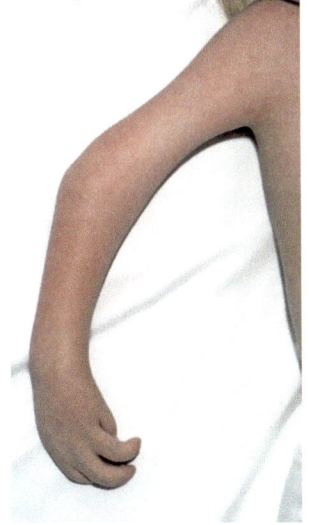

Fig. 7.8 Upper limb in arthrogryposis showing fixed extension of the elbow with only 20° flexion, flexion of the wrist and fingers

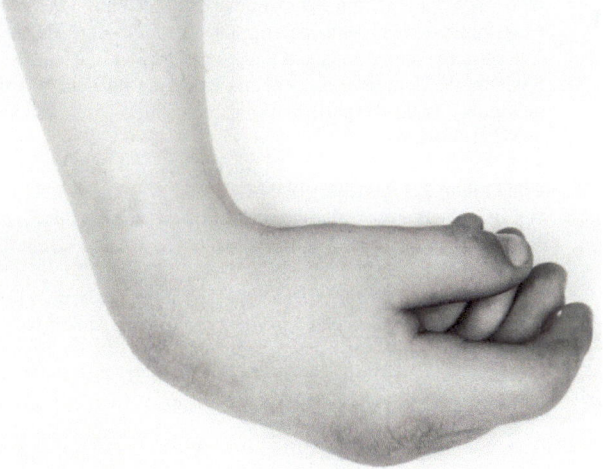

Fig. 7.9 Arthrogrypotic wrist and hand showing typical wrist and finger flexion and adducted thumb

It is extremely difficult to improve finger function because of the basic stiffness of the fingers, and operations are rarely indicated. Release of the thumb adductors and enlargement of the first web space can be useful to correct the "thumb-in-palm" deformity. These patients become extremely adept at using their stiff, flexed fingers and hands as hooks and "hangers," on which articles can be hung and manipulated.

At or near maturity, wrist arthrodesis can be considered both for functional and cosmetic gain but, as in rheumatoid arthritis, it is usually wise to fix the wrist in a slight degree of flexion rather than extension.

Conclusion

These patients cause great distress to their parents when they are born because of their appearance. It is important in the early stages to counsel parents carefully and to be cautious about prognosis until the possible causes of the condition have been elucidated. Those patients who have the classical type of arthrogryposis (amyoplasia congenita) are usually delightful children who are a pleasure to treat because they try so hard and are so adept at finding ways around their physical disabilities. There is a tendency for deformity to recur throughout growth and, as a result, long-term splintage and orthosis are frequently necessary. However, the classical form of the condition is nonprogressive and there is no disorder of sensation, so that the children can benefit significantly from carefully planned surgery and will remain active in adult life.

References

1. Otto AW. Monstrum humanum extremitatibus incurvatus. Monstorum sexcentorum description anatomica in Vratislaviae Museum. Breslau: Anatomico-Pathologieum; 1841:322.
2. Sheldon W. Amyoplasia congenita (multiple congenital articular rigidity: arthrogryposis multiplex congenita). Arch Dis Child 1932; 7:117–136.
3. Hall JG. Genetic aspects of arthrogryposis multiplex congenita. Clin Orthop Rel Res 1985; 194:44–53.
4. Hall JG. Overview of arthrogryposis. In: Staheli LT, Hall JG, Jaffe KM, Pahoike DE, eds. Arthrogryposis: A Text Atlas, Cambridge: Cambridge University Press; 1998:1–25.
5. Hall JG, Reed SD, Green G. The distal arthrogryposis; delineation of new entries: review and nosologic discussion. Am J Med Gen 1982; 11:185–239.
6. Wynne-Davies R, Williams PF, O'Connor JCB. The 1960's epidemic of arthrogryposis multiplex congenita. A survey from the

United Kingdom, Australia and the United States of America. J Bone Joint Surg 1981; 63B:76–82.
7. Bevan WP, Hall JG, Baushad M, Strakeli LJ, et al. Arthrogryposis multiplex congenita (amyoplasia) (An orthopaedic perspective). J Pediatr Orthop 2007; 27:594–598.
8. Palmer PM, MacEwan GD, Bowen JR, Matheus PA. Passive motion therapy for infants with arthrogryposis. Clin Orthop Rel Res 1985; 194:54–59.
9. Robinson RO. Arthrogryposis multiplex congenita: feeding, language and other health problems. Neuropaediatrics 1990; 21: 177–178.
10. Williams PF. Management of upper limb problems in arthrogryposis. Clin Ortho Rel Res 1985; 194:60–67.
11. Robinson RO, Cartwright R, Fixsen JA, Jones M. Arthrogryposis. In: McCarthy GT, ed. Physical Disability in Childhood. Edinburgh, London, New York: Churchill Livingstone; 1992.
12. Green ADL, Fixsen JA, Lloyd-Roberts GC. Talectomy for arthrogryposis multiplex congenita. J Bone Joint Surg 1984; 66B: 697–699.
13. Hsu LCS, Jaffray D, Leong JC. Talectomy for club foot in arthrogryposis. J Bone Joint Surg 1984; 66B:694–696.
14. D'Souza H, Aroojis A, Chawara GS. Talectomy in arthrogryposis: analysis of results. J Pediatr Orthop 1998; 18:760–764.
15. Grill F, Franke J. The Ilizarov distractor for the correction of relapsed or neglected clubfoot. J Bone Joint Surg 1987; 69B: 593–597.
16. Reinke KA, Carpenter CT. Ilizarov applications in the pediatric foot. J Pediatr Orthop 1997; 17:796–802.
17. Murray C, Fixsen JA. Management of knee deformity in classical arthrogryposis multiplex congenita (amyoplasia congenita). J Pediatr Orthop 1997; B6:186–191.
18. Fucs PWWB, Svartman C, Cesar de Assumpcao RM, et al. Quadricepsplasty in arthrogryposis (amyoplasia): Long term follow-up. J Pediatr Orthop 2005; B14:219–224.
19. Parsch K, Pietrazak S. Arthrogryposis multiplex congenital. Orthopade 2007; 36:281–292.
20. Damsin JP, Trousseau A. Treatment of severe flexion deformity of the knee in children and adolescence using the Ilizarov technique. J Bone Joint Surg 1996; 78B:140–144.
21. Brunner R, Hefti F, Tgetgel JC. Arthrogrypotic joint contracture of the knee in children and adolescence using the Ilizarov technique. J Bone Joint Surg 1997; 78B:140–144.
22. Lloyd-Roberts GC, Lettin AWF. Arthrogryposis multiplex congenita. J Bone Joint Surg 1970; 52B:494–508.
23. Staheli LT, Chew ED, Elliott JS, Mosea VS. Management of hip dislocation in children with arthrogryposis. J Pediatr Orthop 1987; 7:681–685.
24. Szoke G, Staheli LT, Jaffe K, Hall JG. Medial approach open reduction of hip dislocation in amyoplasia type arthrogryposis. J Pediatr Orthop 1996; 16:127–130.
25. Akazawa H, Mitani S, Yoshitaka T, et al. Surgical management of hip dislocation in children with arthrogryposis multiplex congenita. J Bone Joint Surg 1998 80B:636–640.
26. Yau PWP, Chow W, Li YH, et al. Twenty year follow-up of hip problems in arthrogryposis multiplex congenital. J Pediatr Orthop 2002; 22:359–363.
27. Axt MW, Niethard FU, Doderlein L, Weber M. Principals of treatment of the upper extremity in arthrogryposis multiplex congenita type 1. J Pediatr Orthop 1997; B6:179–185.
28. Lahoti O, Bell MJ. Transfer of pectoralis major in arthrogryposis to restore elbow function. J Bone Joint Surg 2005; 87B:858–860.

Chapter 8

The Limping Child

F. Stig Jacobsen and Göran Hansson

Introduction

Evaluating a limp in a growing child is a problem often faced by paediatricians, accident and emergency department doctors, general practitioners, and orthopaedic surgeons. There are many causes, ranging from surgical emergencies to children who need observation only [1]. It is often not possible to know with certainty how serious the condition is at the initial examination, and so it is important to adopt a systematic approach to evaluation.

The aim of this chapter is to give an overview of the limping child, to discuss the important points in the history and physical examination, to suggest appropriate imaging and laboratory tests, and to describe the most common causes. Treatment will be dealt with in the relevant chapters.

History

The history of a limp is just as important as the findings on physical examination. If the right questions are asked a provisional diagnosis can be made in most cases at the primary examination. Although the history may be difficult to obtain from a toddler it is usually possible to identify the specific anatomical area involved at the initial examination. The commonest site for symptoms in the limping child is the hip (34%), followed by the knee (19%), the remainder of the leg (18%), and the spine (fewer than 2%) [2]. Most children presenting with a limp have pain [2]. The likelihood of referred pain is greater in children than in adults [3]: pain from the spine may be referred to the thigh or the abdomen and hip pain is very often referred to the thigh or the knee.

The patient's age is important. Fractures and infection are seen in all age groups but some conditions are more age-specific (Table 8.1). Child abuse is most commonly seen in children under the age of 2 years, Legg–Calvé–Perthes' disease between 4 and 8 years, and a slipped capital femoral epiphysis is in adolescence.

A family history, past medical history, and details of previous treatment must be obtained together with an assessment of the child's general health.

The onset of fever should be noted, when it started, its variability, and whether the child is receiving any antipyretic medication or antibiotics. A preceding illness was found by Fischer and Beattie [2] in about 40% of children who presented with an acute limp.

It is important to determine whether the onset of the limp was sudden, as in trauma, or whether it came on gradually,

Table 8.1 Age-Specific Diagnosis of a Limp

Age	Condition
1–3 years	Developmental dysplasia of the hip
	Child abuse
	Tumor
	Neuromuscular disease
	Juvenile idiopathic arthritis
	Leg length discrepancy
	Infections
4–10 years	Transient synovitis
	Legg–Calvé–Perthes disease
	Leg length discrepancy
	Tumor
	Juvenile idiopathic arthritis
	Infections
	Köhler's disease
Greater than 10 years	Slipped capital femoral epiphysis
	Overuse syndrome such as
	Anterior knee pain: Osgood–Schlatter's disease
	Shin splints
	Tarsal coalition
	Heel pain
All age groups	Trauma
	Tumor
	Infection

F.S. Jacobsen (✉)
Orthopaedics Department, Marshfield Clinic, Marshfield, WI, USA

which is typical of chronic disease. A history of trauma or a change in activity may prompt suspicion of a fracture or stress reaction. It is essential to ask about the duration of the limp and any aggravating factors. Juvenile idiopathic arthritis usually presents with limp and stiffness which are more marked in the early morning when the child gets out of bed. Neuromuscular problems are usually worse toward the end of the day because of muscle fatigue. Constant pain during the entire day and night should raise concern about a possible tumor.

Gait

Physical examination should start by observing the child's gait. The physician must therefore be familiar with normal gait patterns and motor development in children (Chapter 6).

Most children under 1 year are able to stand unassisted and cruise and are able to walk before 18 months. The toddler, however, has an immature gait that differs from that of the adult [4] and walks on a broad base in an abrupt and choppy fashion, with a faster cadence (steps/minute) but a slower velocity (cm/second) than the adult.

Fully mature gait is usually attained by 4 years and all subsequent changes in gait are related to change in height [4].

When examining gait the child should be wearing a minimum of clothing and must walk barefooted. Where possible the patient should be seen walking and running unassisted in a large room or a corridor which accentuates any pathological features of gait. To detect muscle weakness it is important to watch the child getting up unaided from the floor and climbing stairs.

The different components of the gait cycle should each receive attention with focus placed sequentially on the feet, the knees, and the hips. Often the child tries to walk normally and the abnormality of gait is seen only when the child thinks he or she is unobserved.

Pathological Gait

A child's limp may be caused by *pain, stiffness, structural change, weakness*, or a combination of these.

Antalgic Gait

The most common limp is antalgic (anti-pain), when the child "hurries off" the affected leg, so limiting the time spent upon it in the stance phase [5]. This is associated with a

shorter swing phase on the opposite leg and a decreased stride length [6]. An antalgic gait can be due to any painful condition such as trauma, transient synovitis, and infection.

If the spine is affected the child walks carefully and slowly avoiding trunk rotation that exacerbates pain.

Leg Length Discrepancy Gait

The patient with a leg length discrepancy compensates either by walking on tiptoe on the short side or with slight hip and knee flexion on the long side, in an endeavor to balance leg length.

Trendelenburg Gait

A Trendelenburg gait is a painless limp in a patient with either weak hip abductor muscles or an unstable hip fulcrum. In the stance phase, the opposite side of the pelvis drops. To compensate, the child leans over the affected hip. Bilateral involvement causes a waddling gait with a bilateral lurch. The time spent in the stance phase on the affected leg is normal, as pain is often absent. A typical Trendelenburg gait is seen in developmental dysplasia of the hip or in those hip problems in which overgrowth of the greater trochanter weakens the hip abductors.

Gait in Cerebral Palsy

The gait pattern in cerebral palsy depends on the specific brain lesion, secondary muscle contractures, and compensatory movements (see Chapters 6 and 19). Tightness in the gastrocnemius–soleus complex and the hamstrings often causes toe walking and secondary flexion of the knee during stance. Rotational malalignment of femur or tibia leads to in or out toeing and tight adductors to scissoring. Relative weakness of the gastrocnemius–soleus complex causes a typical crouched gait, with increased flexion of the hips and the knees. A spastic rectus femoris muscle can give rise to a stiff knee gait, with difficulties of foot clearance during the swing phase.

Gait in Muscular Dystrophy

The muscle weakness in many muscular dystrophy patients causes a very characteristic posture and gait (see Chapter 16). Duchenne's muscular dystrophy, with early and striking proximal hip extensor weakness, causes hip flexion contractures and a secondary lumbar lordosis which brings the centre of gravity over the hip. The child tiptoes because of tightness and early contracture of the gastrocnemius–soleus complex with a wide, waddling Trendelenburg gait.

Physical Examination

Standing

With the patient standing the back should be examined for scoliosis, local tenderness, and range of motion. The whole spine must be visible. If a pelvic tilt is present it can be corrected by placing blocks under the shorter leg until the pelvis is level. A positive Trendelenburg test may indicate hip dysplasia, the sequelae of Legg–Calvé–Perthes' disease, or slipped capital femoral epiphysis. Spine motion should be tested as it will be limited with discitis and extension will be painful with spondylolysis.

Cutaneous changes such as skin dimples and hairy patches over the lumbar spine, erythema, or heat over joints should be noted. Café au lait spots, particularly in the axillae, should lead to the suspicion of neurofibromatosis or fibrous dysplasia.

Supine

With the patient supine each joint should be examined separately. Look for swelling, feel for tenderness, and assess movement. Hip flexion contracture can be judged by Thomas's test. The abdomen should always be examined, as conditions such as appendicitis can occasionally present as a limp [7].

A full neurological examination should be performed to assess atrophy, muscle strength and tone, sensation, and reflexes. Atrophy of the quadriceps muscle is often associated with a painful hip or knee and correlates with the duration of symptoms.

The examiner should check for leg length discrepancy by measuring the distance from the anterior superior spine to the medial malleolus, in addition to examining the patient standing to look for a pelvic tilt. A short leg must be distinguished from apparent shortening that is caused by scoliosis with pelvic obliquity or joint contracture. Rarely the longer leg, whether true or apparent, is the abnormal one.

Prone

Hip rotation in extension is best tested with the patient prone. The knees are flexed to 90 and the tibiae used as lever arms. The amount of internal and external rotation can easily be measured and any asymmetry detected. Limited painful internal rotation of the hip suggests synovitis of the hip joint or a slipped capital femoral epiphysis. Further, with the patient prone, femoral anteversion can be measured and tibial torsion evaluated by measuring the foot–thigh angle.

Diagnostic Investigations

Blood Tests

Most of these are nonspecific. Appropriate tests depend on the patient's history and physical examination. Any patient with fever or possible infection should have a complete blood count, white blood count, erythrocyte sedimentation rate (ESR), and C-reactive protein (CRP) tests performed. Blood cultures are important and should ideally be taken at fever peaks.

An ESR of 50 mm/h or more strongly suggests serious disease in children who present with a limp [8]. The C-reactive protein concentration usually increases and subsequently decreases more rapidly than the ESR. It is, therefore, more useful for assessing the efficacy of treatment [9]. In children in whom an arthritic etiology is suspected, rheumatoid factor, antinuclear antibodies, HLA B27, and Lyme titre should be checked, although many of these may be negative in the early stages of the disease.

Joint Aspiration

Joint effusions should always be aspirated when infection is suspected. The aspirate should be sent for Gram staining, aerobic and anaerobic culture, a cell count, and glucose determination (compared with blood glucose levels).

Diagnostic Imaging

Plain Radiographs

These are readily accessible, inexpensive, and specific for a whole range of disorders such as tumor, infection, or fracture [10] (see Chapter 5). Although they give information on bone pathology they may not show early changes and give limited information about soft tissue and cartilage. There are many conditions, therefore, not detectable by radiograph alone [11].

Simple radiological examination should be undertaken first. An anteroposterior and a lateral view are always necessary. A comparative view of the contralateral limb is often useful. Specific radiographs may be necessary (e.g., oblique radiographs of the lumbar spine may show a pars interarticularis defect; a lateral view of the hip is always necessary in suspected slipped capital femoral epiphysis; a tunnel view for osteochondritis dissecans of the knee; oblique radiographs of the foot to show calcaneonavicular coalition).

Bone Scintigraphy

This uses a tracer, technetium-99m-labeled methylene diphosphate, which is concentrated in areas of osteoblastic activity. It is a nonspecific test that highlights areas of increased bone metabolism.

Bone scintigraphy may detect subtle abnormalities such as stress fractures before they are evident on plain radiograph. It cannot differentiate between different diseases but helps to indicate the anatomical area involved [12]. Aronson et al. [13] found bone scans of great value in a group of limping children in whom the diagnosis was in doubt.

A bone scan need not always show increased activity to be positive. A photon-deficient (cold) scan may be seen in osteomyelitis, particularly in the neonate. The rapid progression of bacterial infection in bone and subperiosteum can cause increased intraosseous pressure and decreased blood flow. Affected patients have aggressive osteomyelitis and need urgent treatment [14].

Ultrasound Imaging

Ultrasound of the hip shows the relationship of the cartilaginous femoral head to the acetabulum. It also offers dynamic evaluation of hip stability without irradiation. The child does not require sedation.

Ultrasound is invaluable in assessing hip effusions and synovitis, as seen in transient synovitis, Legg–Calvé–Perthes' disease, or juvenile idiopathic arthritis. The normal hip capsule appears concave but, with an effusion, it balloons out and becomes convex. A 2-mm separation between the femoral neck and the joint capsule is diagnostic (Fig. 8.1) [15].

Ultrasonography is very useful in checking for an effusion in all limb joints. Early subperiosteal collections of fluid or pus in osteomyelitis are detectable well before lamellar new bone can be seen on radiograph. It also helps to guide aspiration.

Computed Tomography (CT)

This determines more precisely the anatomy of an area involved and is particularly useful in osteoid osteoma, in evaluating a tarsal coalition or the patellofemoral joint and, of course, in some tumors.

Magnetic Resonance Imaging

Magnetic resonance imaging (MRI) is an expensive and highly sophisticated tool capable of providing a great deal of information. It can be useful in the early diagnosis of Legg–Calvé–Perthes' disease, avascular necrosis, and in the assessment of tumors and infections. However, most young children will require sedation or anesthesia.

Causes of Limping

Trauma is by far the most common reason for a child to limp. The etiology of non-traumatic causes of limping varies, but is often inflammatory (Table 8.2). In one review, 23% of

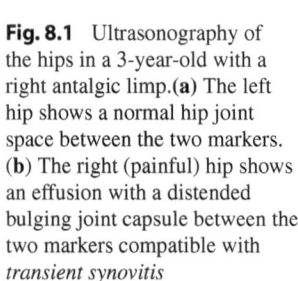

Fig. 8.1 Ultrasonography of the hips in a 3-year-old with a right antalgic limp.(**a**) The left hip shows a normal hip joint space between the two markers. (**b**) The right (painful) hip shows an effusion with a distended bulging joint capsule between the two markers compatible with *transient synovitis*

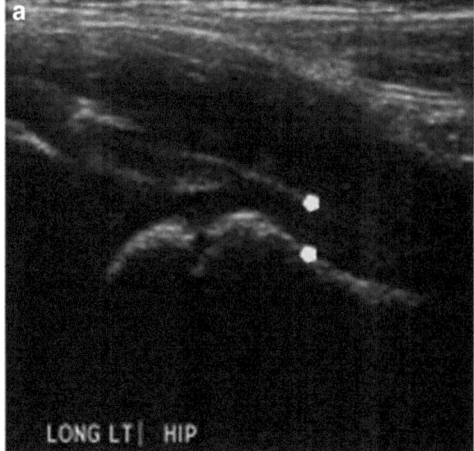
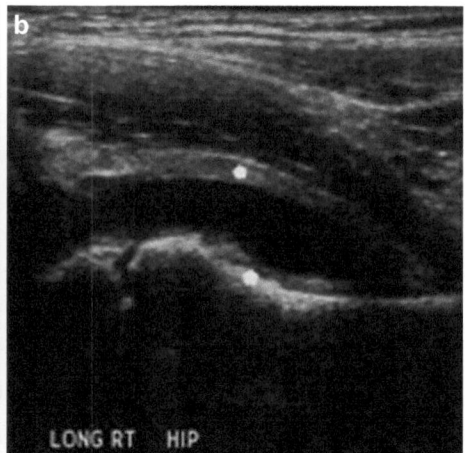

Table 8.2 Differential diagnosis of acute atraumatic limp after Fischer & Beattie [2]

Cause	Frequency in %
Inflammatory	
Tansient synovitis	39,5
Juvenile arthritis, viral illness	3,2
Infection	3,6
Developmental or acquired (LCP, SUFE etc)	4,1
Neoplasia	0,8
Muscle strain, overuse	17,7
Others (torsion of testis, orchitis etc)	1,2
No definite diagnosis made	29,9
	100,0

children younger than 5 years who presented with a limp or refusal to bear weight proved to have a severe bacterial infection [16].

In the differential diagnosis of acute limp without obvious trauma the majority is caused by transient synovitis. In almost 30% of children a definite diagnosis could not be found. (Table 8.2)

Trauma

Fractures

They are usually apparent clinically and radiologically. They require appropriate treatment by reduction if necessary and immobilization.

A toddler tibial fracture is a common reason for limping. It is a low energy, usually non-displaced, fracture of the tibia without concomitant fibula fracture. The parents often do not recall trauma. The child presents with a limp or refusal to weight bear. The initial radiograph is often negative but follow-up radiographs a week or two later usually show the fracture or periosteal elevation (Fig. 8.2). Treatment consists of a cast immobilization. Similarly in the toddler a fracture of the calcaneus may be difficult to diagnose and to see on plain radiographs unless an axial view is taken.

Stress Fractures

These are a common cause of limping in children, especially in adolescence. When seen in otherwise normal bone they are the result of increased or repetitive muscle action rather than direct impact [17]. Bone responds to excessive stress by remodeling and resorption and eventually by increased bone formation. A stress fracture develops when the fatigue process exceeds the bone repair process.

Fractures may also occur as a result of normal physiological stresses in bones with deficient elastic resistance [17]. These insufficiency fractures may occur in bone tumors,

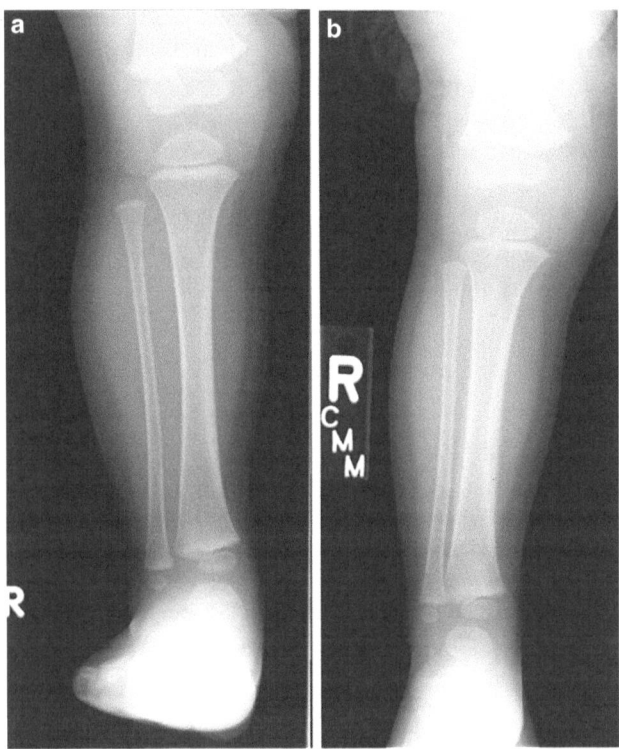

Fig. 8.2 (**a**) Normal radiograph of an 18-month-old boy with a limp and slight tenderness of the lower tibia. He was treated in a cast on suspicion of a fracture. (**b**) Radiograph 2 weeks later showing the periosteal elevation typical of a healing *toddler's fracture*

osteogenesis imperfecta, rickets, or the osteoporosis associated with immobilization or cerebral palsy. Anatomical conditions may also predispose to stress fracture; for instance a rigid cavus or flat foot may fail to absorb energy normally.

The most common site for a stress fracture is the tibia, which accounts for up to 50% of all cases [18]. The fractures, which occur most frequently in 10–15-year-olds, are usually located between the metaphysis and diaphysis of the proximal tibia, either on the posteromedial or on the posterolateral corner. The fibula is the second most common site of stress fracture, usually in a younger age group. Stress fractures also occur in the metatarsals, calcaneum, pelvis, and femur (see Chapter 38).

Stress fractures are most common in younger children in spring, when activity levels increase after an inactive winter. In the adolescent, when the bone elasticity of the young is decreasing, stress fractures develop during or after athletic activities.

Symptoms depend on the stress fracture site but the most common complaint is pain related to activity, relieved by rest, and associated with an antalgic gait. Local swelling and tenderness may be present. There is often a history of increased or changed activity or a change of shoes or running surface. Radiographs initially show a small cortical lucency followed by a gradual increase in periosteal and endosteal bone formation. These findings may take up to 3 weeks to appear depending on the patient's age.

A bone scan is useful in the early detection of a stress fracture before other radiological changes occur. MRI and CT may help to establish the diagnosis in difficult cases. The differential diagnoses include tumors such as osteoid osteoma and Ewing's sarcoma. Biopsy can be misleading because the changes of fracture repair may be hard to differentiate from a tumor.

Fig. 8.3 Lateral knee radiograph of 12-year-old boy with a painful limp and tenderness over the distal patellar pole. The small avulsion at the inferior pole represents *Sinding–Larsen–Johansson disease*

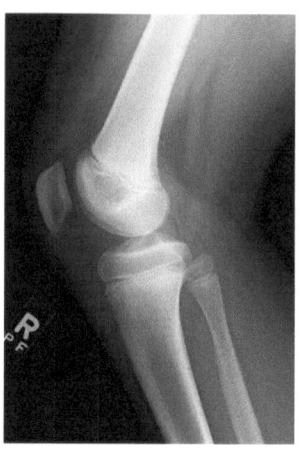

Overuse Syndromes

Increasing numbers of children now participate in organized sport. This increase is matched by the numbers who present with overuse syndromes, often with a painful limp. Overuse injuries often occur where tendons, ligaments, muscles, and bone adjoin. Children who have recently undergone a significant growth spurt have less flexibility and are more prone to injury.

The following overuse syndromes may cause a limp:

1. *Spondylolysis* is a stress fracture of the pars interarticularis common in sports such as gymnastics, rowing, diving, weightlifting, bowling, and throwing.
2. *Iliac apophysitis* may be seen in adolescent runners. It is also called a "hip pointer" and presents with pain over the iliac crest one hands breadth behind the anterior superior iliac spine [19]. Avulsion of a pelvic apophysis may follow violent contraction of the hamstrings, adductors, or the iliopsoas and is common in jumping and sprinting. Pain and tenderness are localized in the groin or buttock and the diagnosis is confirmed by radiograph. Non-weight-bearing with crutches is usually the only treatment necessary.
3. *Osgood–Schlatter's disease* is the most common condition around the knee. It is a stress-related partial avulsion injury of the tibial tubercle, with inflammatory changes and swelling. It occurs most commonly in boys between 10 and 15 years, with symptoms of local pain, swelling, and discomfort with activity. Radiographs show soft tissue swelling and fragmentation of the tibial tubercle.
4. *Sinding–Larsen–Johansson disease* causes anterior knee pain and is probably caused by excessive and repetitive traction on the inferior pole of the patella. It is also seen in patients with cerebral palsy and a "crouch gait." There is usually striking tenderness of the inferior pole of the patella (Fig. 8.3).

5. *Patellofemoral pain* is common in girls and often occurs in association with increased femoral anteversion, knee valgus, external tibial torsion, etc. It may or may not be associated with patellar instability and tracking needs to be carefully checked.
6. *Sever's disease* (Haglund's disease) is characterized by pain and tenderness at the tendo Achilles insertion into the calcaneal apophysis. It is usually chronic and related to activity. Although plain radiographs may show fragmentation of the calcaneal apophysis this may be a normal finding in this age group and is nonspecific.

When an overuse syndrome is correctly diagnosed, treatment is usually pain control and activity modification followed by rehabilitation.

Child Abuse

This must be considered when a child is in pain or limps with no clear cause, particularly if the child is younger than 2 years. It should be considered in a child with a questionable history of trauma or a delay in presenting to the physician. It is important to look for other manifestations such as bruises and burns. The matter is considered in more detail in Chapter 42.

No single lesion is specific for child abuse but certain fracture patterns are suggestive. Fractures before walking age, metaphyseal corner fractures, and multiple fractures at different stages of healing should all alert concern. Spiral fractures of the humerus, femur, and tibia, together with inexplicable rib fractures, should prompt a search for others by skeletal survey. If abuse is suspected the abuse team must be notified. It is, of course, important to rule out other causes of fracture such as fibrous dysplasia, osteogenesis imperfecta.

Inflammatory Synovitis

Transient Synovitis of The Hip

Transient synovitis is the most common cause of hip pain in children [20]. Synonyms include "irritable hip," "observation hip," and "coxalgia fugax." It is a noninfective synovitis characterized by a sudden onset of hip pain and limp in a child who is not systemically ill. Children, more commonly boys, aged 3–8 years are the most vulnerable. The accumulated risk of suffering transient synovitis before 14 years has been shown to be 3% [21]. Repeated episodes occur in 10%, usually within 6 months of the first episode [22].

Etiology

The cause is unknown but trauma, infection, and allergy have been implicated. An infectious etiology is supported by the finding that children have often had a preceding viral upper respiratory tract infection and that the synovitis is seen most often in the autumn, when the incidence of viral infection is high.

Clinical Findings

The child may present with only a limp but may complain of pain in hip, thigh, or knee. Hip movement may vary from slightly to very considerably restricted and some children cannot bear weight.

The patient is usually afebrile but may have a temperature of up to 38–39°C without being systemically ill. The hip joint is typically held in flexion and abduction to accommodate an effusion in the joint. Internal rotation of the hip is limited and painful, the most consistent finding in transient synovitis and is best looked for with the patient prone [23].

The synovitis commonly lasts for only a few days and there is usually complete resolution of the symptoms. The long-term effects of transient synovitis are probably benign [24]. In a long-term follow-up of 23 patients De Valderrama [25] found that up to 50% developed coxa magna, with a slight risk of developing arthritis in the involved hip. However, 67% of his patients spent 3–5 months in hospital, which suggests a more severe disorder than our present concept of "transient synovitis."

It has been postulated that transient synovitis is a precursor of Legg–Calvé–Perthes' disease [26]. Kallio et al. [27], however, found no case of Legg–Calvé–Perthes' disease after 1 year in their study of 119 children with transient synovitis. They suggest that cases described in the literature were examples of early stage Legg–Calvé–Perthes'. While some recommend a radiograph of the hip 3 months after the synovitis to exclude Legg–Calvé–Perthes', this is not justified in the asymptomatic child.

Investigations

Conventional *radiographs* are normal in typical transient synovitis. Apparent capsular distension and lost fat planes depend on rotation of the leg and are not true indicators of an effusion.

Ultrasound is the method of choice for diagnosing a joint effusion. Intracapsular synovitis and fluid can be directly visualized and measured. The child is positioned supine with the leg in the neutral position. Anterior ultrasonography shows the distance between the femoral neck and the anterior joint capsule (Fig. 8.1). A full blood count, ESR, and CRP may reassure that there is no infection.

Treatment

This is symptomatic, resting in bed with the hip flexed or non-weight-bearing with crutches and anti-inflammatory medication. Unless infection is suspected children should not need hospital admission. When the hip is very irritable, an ultrasound-guided hip aspiration allows the synovial fluid to be analyzed for infection and swiftly relieves discomfort.

Differential Diagnosis

It may be difficult to distinguish transient synovitis from other hip disorders. Early Legg–Calvé–Perthes' disease is clinically similar to transient synovitis. Initial radiographic changes in Legg–Calvé–Perthes' may be subtle. When in doubt a bone scan or MRI may help to distinguish them.

Juvenile idiopathic arthritis, if seronegative, may initially be difficult to diagnose, but the insidious onset and protracted course serve to distinguish it.

Other diagnoses to be considered include osteoid osteoma of the proximal femur with reactive synovitis, slipped capital femoral epiphysis in its early stages, or bone or soft tissue infections in the pelvis. Plain radiographs are rarely diagnostic and MRI or bone scintigraphy may be useful (Fig. 8.4).

The critical differential diagnosis of transient synovitis is *septic arthritis,* which may need urgent drainage and systemic antibiotics. The clinical findings may be similar, but a high temperature is uncommon in transient synovitis. In one study, 97% of children with septic arthritis had an ESR greater than 20 mm/h, a temperature of more than 37.5°C, or both [28]. There is, however, an overlap in the parameters and in the same study 47% of the patients with transient synovitis

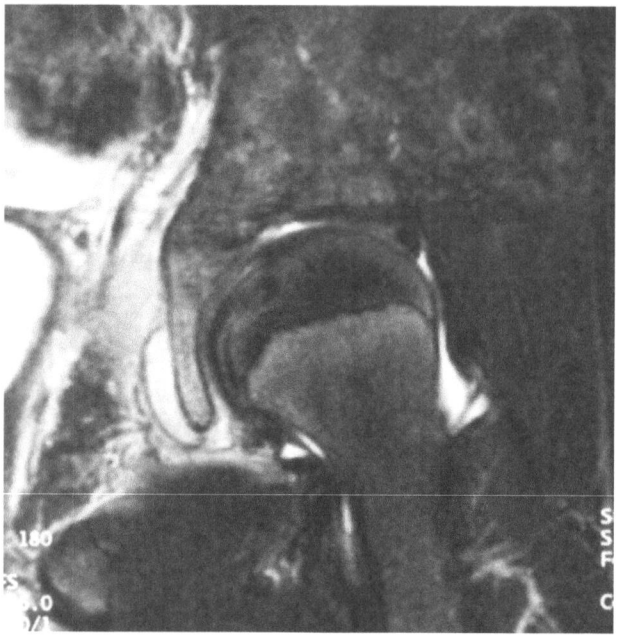

Fig. 8.4 MRI of an 11-year-old with a limp and a temperature of 38°C. There was slight tenderness over the left hip but normal movement. Radiographs and ultrasound images were normal but the MRI shows an *abscess on the inner side of the acetabulum*

Table 8.3 Four-parameter* assessment for septic arthritis [29]

Number of parameters present	Probability for septic arthritis (%)
0	0.2
1	3.0
2	40.0
3	93.1
4	99.6

*Fever >38.5°; non-weight-bearing; ESR > 40 mm/h; white blood count > 12,000 cells/mm^3

had similar positive parameters. The C-reactive protein value guides the clinician better but the general rule is that any child with a fever and an increased ESR should be suspected of having septic arthritis.

In one study Kocher et al. [29] considered four independent parameters to distinguish between the two entities (Table 8.3).

The consequences of overlooking septic arthritis can be devastating: patients with two or more positive parameters should have the affected joint aspirated.

Juvenile Idiopathic Arthritis

This generalized systemic arthritis differs from adult rheumatoid arthritis in both course and prognosis. Subgroups are described on the basis of joint involvement and systemic disease. The condition is considered in detail in Chapter 13.

Juvenile idiopathic arthritis often presents with single joint involvement. The onset is usually gradual and less severe than that seen in infection. If the lower extremity is involved, the child may present with an antalgic limp, joint swelling, and slight discomfort. The diagnosis is often made by exclusion and blood tests may help. If the joint is aspirated the cell count is usually 2,000–50,000 cells/mm^3 range, whereas in infection the count usually exceeds 50,000.

Reactive Arthritis

This describes a systemic disease not limited to joints alone, despite its name. Reactive arthritis is a response to infection elsewhere in the body, such as the upper airway, gastrointestinal, or urogenital tracts. It is probably autoimmune and results from a crossover reaction between synovial and infectious antigens. The knee, ankle, or hip is usually involved and the patient feels unwell and feverish. The arthritis develops acutely with severe pain and there is often a migratory polyarthritis. If the condition follows a group A streptococcal pharyngitis it can be diagnosed by the presence of an antibody response to group A streptococcus, usually 1–2 weeks after the infection.

The clinical presentation can mimic septic arthritis [30] and may warrant joint aspiration. The joint fluid is sterile but the white blood cell count in the joint fluid is frequently increased.

The reactive arthritis group of diseases merges with others such as Reiter's syndrome and ankylosing spondylitis. In the spondyloarthropathies, the sacroiliac joint is frequently involved and peripheral joint symptoms occur in most children. An enthesopathy, with pain and tenderness at tendon–bone junctions, offers an early diagnostic clue. The inflammation at these sites is often striking and causes a significant limp. The strong association with a positive HLA B27 suggests a genetic factor. Reactive arthritis may also follow acute rheumatic fever and enteric infections from bacteria such as *Shigella*, *Salmonella*, and *Yersinia*.

Virus infections may also give rise to reactive arthritis or arthralgia. This usually lasts for 1–2 weeks and may be migratory. It may follow rubella infection or immunization, alphavirus infection, or herpes virus infection.

Reactive arthritis is often a diagnosis of exclusion.

Infections

Osteomyelitis

Osteomyelitis occurs at any age in childhood (see Chapter 10) and is caused by the hematological spread of bacteria which usually seed in the metaphyses of long bones, especially those of the femur, the pelvis, and the tibia [31]. Osteomyelitis of the pelvis or upper femur is often adjacent to the hip and can present with hip pain and gait disturbance [32]. Established infections in bone can spread into the adjacent joint, either through the epiphysis in very young children or in the hip, directly from the intracapsular metaphysis. It is important always to examine adjacent joints, as 30% of patients have associated septic joint involvement [33].

Pelvic osteomyelitis presents with fever, pain, and limping. There may be localized tenderness. Most patients have pain and reduced hip movement, which is less marked than in septic arthritis of the hip. If the abscess is located in the obturator internus muscle it can easily be mistaken for septic arthritis of the hip (see Fig. 8.4) [34]. Radiographic changes develop late and ultrasound, MRI, or bone scan allow much earlier diagnosis.

Subacute osteomyelitis is becoming more common. The patient often presents with a painful limp but the diagnosis is frequently delayed as the symptoms develop slowly, the patient is afebrile, and laboratory tests are often normal (Fig. 8.5).

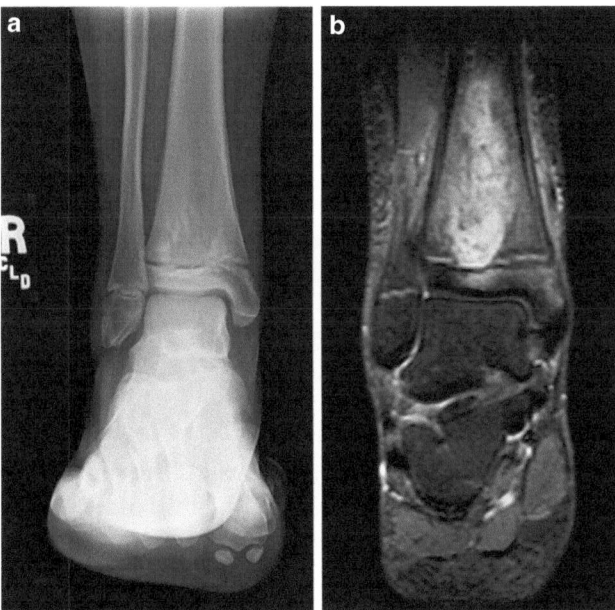

Fig. 8.5 (**a**) Radiograph of a 14-year-old boy's ankle showing a lytic lesion in the distal tibial metaphysis. He gave a 7-week history of a limp and pain but had no fever and only slight tenderness. (**b**) MRI shows the lesion crossing the physis with some edema in the epiphysis. Surgery confirmed *subacute osteomyelitis*

Septic Arthritis

Prompt, accurate diagnosis is essential to allow early treatment and obtain optimal results (see Chapter 10). Septic arthritis of the hip, knee, and ankle account for more than 90% of all cases [1.]

The patient is usually febrile, with a temperature greater than 38°C, and presents with a painful joint that is warm and red with limited, painful movement. In early childhood the fever can be absent or mild. The child who has received antibiotics or is immunodeficient may lack typical symptoms and signs. If the hip joint is involved it is held flexed, abducted, and externally rotated. All movement is restricted and pain may give rise to "pseudoparalysis," especially in infants. Groin or proximal thigh swelling will often be present.

The differential diagnoses include transient synovitis, juvenile idiopathic arthritis, osteomyelitis, Lyme disease, Legg–Calvé–Perthes' disease, and slipped capital femoral epiphysis. Plain radiographs are usually normal in early septic arthritis, although subtle subluxation of the hip occurs early in infants. Even osteomyelitis may be radiologically invisible for many days. The definitive test for septic arthritis of any joint is aspiration, usually guided by ultrasound.

In infection, the joint fluid is usually cloudy with a cell count of more than 50,000 cells/mm^3, most being polymorphonuclear cells. In joint infection and acute rheumatoid arthritis, the synovial fluid glucose level is characteristically lowered. Bacteriological culture is positive in only 30–80%. Patients with negative cultures run a clinical course similar to those with positive cultures and should receive the same aggressive treatment [35].

The treatment of septic arthritis in the hip is immediate open drainage and irrigation. It should be regarded as an orthopaedic emergency, because of the possible severe sequelae. These include avascular necrosis of the femoral head, subluxation or dislocation, and growth plate injury. A good outcome depends on prompt decompression. Complications are more frequent in infants under 6 months old, when treatment is delayed for more than 2–3 days and with adjacent osteomyelitis of the proximal femur. The knee and ankle must be treated depending on disease duration and the response to antibiotics, with repeat aspirations, arthroscopic drainage, or arthrotomy.

Discitis

This disc space disease ranges from a benign self-limiting inflammation to a true osteomyelitis involving adjacent bone [36]. It is usually seen in younger children aged 2–6 years (see Chapter 35). The cause of infection is probably bacterial but may, in milder cases, be viral.

The young child usually presents with a limp or refusal to walk or sit, whereas in the older child back or neck pain is more common. If the patient is walking the gait is stiff and guarded.

Physical examination shows a rigid spine with loss of the lumbar lordosis, muscle spasm, and limited straight leg-raising. The ESR and white blood count are usually increased. Plain radiographs are negative in the first 3–6 weeks of the disease but disc space narrowing and erosion of the vertebral bodies may develop later. Bone scintigraphy may help but MRI seems more reliable in establishing an early diagnosis. MRI is probably the best imaging modality for any child with inexplicable back pain.

Pyogenic sacroiliitis may present as back or hip pain and the patient may have a limp [37]. An epidural abscess can, in the early stages, present in a similar fashion [38].

Psoas Abscess

A psoas abscess is uncommon in countries where tuberculosis is no longer endemic but may occur with infections of the spine or abdomen. The child has a painful limp and a hip flexion contracture. Psoas contracture may be seen following an intramuscular bleed in hemophilia or in patients on anticoagulants. Diagnosis is helped by ultrasound and MRI [39].

Lyme Disease

Lyme disease is caused by the spirochete *Borrelia burgdorferi* and is transmitted to humans by the bite of an infected tick.

While presentation varies greatly, the first sign is usually a circular rash—erythema migrans that appears in 75%. It appears from a few days to a month after the tick bite and can expand with a central clear zone giving a "bull's eye" appearance.

Early manifestations include fatigue, fever, cardiac irregularity, and Bell's palsy, with arthritis and polyneuropathy as later signs. Arthritis, however, can be an early sign and the disease should always be considered in areas where it is endemic [40]. Large joints such as the knee, ankle, or hip are usually affected and the symptoms and signs may resemble pauciarticular juvenile arthritis.

If an effusion is present, aspiration for diagnostic purposes is recommended as there is a considerable overlap in the clinical and laboratory presentation of Lyme disease and septic arthritis [41].

There are three types of antibody tests used to diagnose Lyme disease: enzyme-linked immunosorbent assay (ELISA), indirect fluorescent antibody (IFA), and the western blot test. The most commonly used is the ELISA, which is the most sensitive and rapid test; however, the western blot

test is the most specific and used to detect chronic Lyme disease. Most patients with acute Lyme disease can be treated successfully with a short course of oral antibiotics such as doxycycline, amoxicillin, or cefuroxime. Patients with cardiac or neurological involvement or chronic disease may need a longer period of treatment.

Other Causes of a Limp

Many common childhood hip problems present with a limp. A simple but valuable observation is that a healthy child with a limp should, until proven otherwise, be assumed to have hip dysplasia if younger than 4 years, Legg–Calvé–Perthes' disease if 4–9 years old, and a slipped upper femoral epiphysis if older than 9 years. These are discussed in detail in Chapters 26, 27, and 28, respectively.

Many "knee" symptoms are referred from the hip but there are mechanical disorders of the knee that cause a child to limp. These include patellar instability, dislocations, and osteochondrotic lesions (Chapter 29). Because the growth plates around the knee contribute most to growth, they are the most vulnerable to benign and malignant tumors.

At the foot and ankle, limping in an otherwise healthy child may be caused by osteochondritis dissecans, typically of the talar dome. Recurrent sprains, limping, and peroneal spasm with exercise are complications of a tarsal coalition. Osteochondritis of the navicular (Köhler's disease) and osteochondrosis of the head of the second metatarsal (Freiberg's disease) present with a limp and localized pain and tenderness. It is well to remember also that limping is sometimes caused by a foreign body in either the shoe or the soft tissues of the foot. Pseudomonas infection should be suspected if the child was wearing sneakers at the time of a puncture injury to the foot [42].

Köhler's disease is an avascular necrosis of the tarsal navicular, seen mainly in boys 3–8 years. Patients present with a limp and pain over the medial arch of the foot with local tenderness. Radiographs show a small sclerotic navicular. Fragmentation may be seen but in the absence of symptoms this is a normal variant.

Tumors

Fisher and Beattie [2] reported tumors as the cause of a limp in fewer than 1% of children. However, the possibility must be borne in mind as the consequences of a "missed" or late diagnosis can be very serious (see Chapter 14).

It is important to remember that the tumor causing a painful limp may not be in the lower extremity or pelvis: cerebral and spinal cord tumors may present with a limp [43].

Two tumors that often present with a limp are leukemia and osteoid osteoma. Patients with suspected tumors should

Fig. 8.6 Radiographs of a 7-year-old girl with a limp and right tibial tenderness. (**a**) Plain radiograph shows posterolateral cortical tibial thickening. (**b**) Bone scintigraphy shows increased uptake in the distal tibia. (**c**) CT scan illustrates a typical *osteoid osteoma*

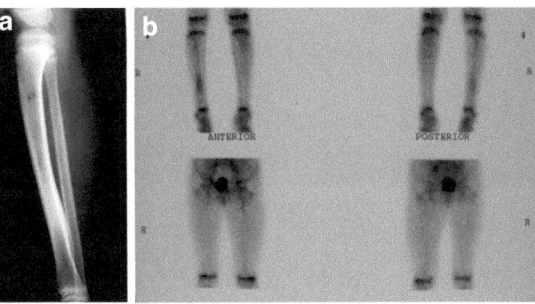
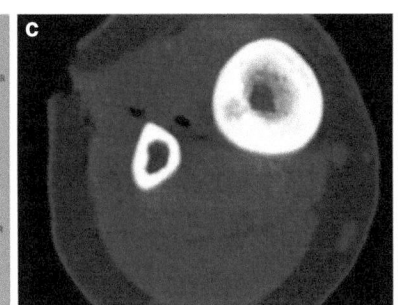

have anteroposterior and lateral radiographs performed. Further studies such as bone scintigraphy, CT, and MRI will usually be necessary both for diagnosis and to stage the tumor.

Leukemia

Leukemia is the commonest childhood malignancy and may present at any age. The orthopaedic surgeon may see the patient first as some will present with a limp [44]. Clinical signs are vague but include fever, lethargy, bruising, and infection. Bone aches and joint pains are frequent and often present asymmetrically in the hips or knees. The symptoms may resemble those of juvenile idiopathic arthritis.

Radiological signs are nonspecific and include osteoporosis, periosteal reaction, sclerosis, or lytic lesions. Metaphyseal lucencies (leukemic lines) are often the first radiological change, commonly around the knee. However, this banding is nonspecific and can be seen also in malnutrition, juvenile idiopathic arthritis, and septicemia. Bone pain is caused by the proliferation of hemopoietic tissue within the medullary canal and may occur without any obvious radiological changes.

The patient will have anemia, thrombocytopenia, and an increased ESR. Surprisingly, about 50% have a low leucocyte count. The diagnosis is confirmed by bone marrow aspiration.

Osteoid Osteoma

This presents as a painful bone lesion in children usually over the age of 5 years. Most lesions are located in the lower limbs but can occur elsewhere (e.g., in the spine); the child presents with pain and a limp. Pain occurs after activity and typically at night, when it is relieved by aspirin.

There may be tenderness, increased warmth, and swelling if the tumor is superficial. The diagnosis can sometimes be made on plain radiographs, where periosteal thickening and endosteal sclerosis are seen. Bone scintigraphy shows increased uptake, but the nidus is best visualized with a CT scan (Fig. 8.6).

Fig. 8.7 Radiograph of the right hip of a 15-year-old boy who had limped for several months. The large lytic lesion in the femoral neck and greater trochanter was shown at biopsy to be an *aneurysmal bone cyst*

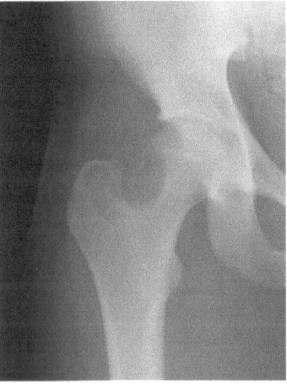

Histiocytosis-X (Langerhans' Cell Histiocytosis [LCH])

Eosinophil granuloma is the commonest of these. If in the lower extremity, it can cause pain and a limp. Spinal involvement may lead to vertebral body collapse (vertebra plana). There may be systemic upset in which case up to 20% may have pulmonary involvement.

Radiograph shows a lytic destructive lesion with a periosteal reaction which may mimic other tumors. CT scans and MRI may help but an unequivocal diagnosis can only be made by biopsy.

Bone Cysts

Unicameral bone cysts or aneurysmal bone cysts may present with a complete fracture or with a limp due to microfracture. The diagnosis is frequently not be made until a fracture occurs (Fig. 8.7).

References

1. Lawrence LL. The limping child. Emerg Med Clin North Am 1998; 16:4:911–929.
2. Fischer SU, Beattie TF. The limping child: Epidemiology, Assessment and Outcome. J Bone Joint Surg 1999; 81B 1029–1034.

3. Hensinger RN. Limp. Pediatr Clin North Am 1986; 33: 6:1355–1362.

4. Sutherland D. The development of mature gait. Gait Posture 1997; 6:163–170.

5. Dabney KW, Lipton G. Evaluation of limp in children. Curr Opinion Pediat 1995; 7:88–94.

6. Phillips WA. The child with a limp. Orthop Clin North Am 1987; 18:4:489–501.

7. Renshaw TS. The child who has a limp. Pediatr Rev 1995; 16: 12:458–465.

8. Huttenlocher A, Newman TB. Evaluation of the erythrocyte sedimentation rate in children presenting with limp, fever or abdominal pain. Clin Pediatr 1997; 339–344.

9. Unkila-Kallio L, Kallio MJT, Eskola J, Peltola, H. Serum C-reactive protein, erythrocyte sedimentation rate and white blood cell count in acute hematogenous osteomyelitis of children. Pediatrics 1994; 93:59–62.

10. Myers MT, Thompson GH. Imaging the child with a limp. Pediatr Clin North Am 1997; 44:3:637–658.

11. Blatt SD, Rosenthal BM, Barnhart, DC. Diagnostic utility of lower extremity radiographs of young children with gait disturbance. Pediatrics 1991; 87:138–140.

12. Connolly LP, Treves ST. Assessing the limping child with skeletal scintigraphy. J Nucl Med. 1998; 39:6:1056–1061.

13. Aronson J, Garvin K, Seibert J, et al. Efficiency of the bone scan for occult limping toddlers. J Pediatr Orthop 1992; 12: 38–44.

14. Pennington WT, Mott MP, Thometz JG, et al. Photopenic bone scan osteomyelitis: a clinical perspective. J Pediatr Orthop 1999; 19:695–698.

15. Terjesen T, Osthus P. Ultrasound in the diagnosis and follow-up of transient synovitis of the hip. J Pediatr Orthop 1991; 11:608–613.

16. Choban S, Killian JT. Evaluation of acute gait abnormalities in preschool children. J Pediatr Orthop 1990; 10:74–78.

17. Ogden JA. Skeletal Injury in a Child. Philadelphia: Lee & Febiger. 1982.

18. Walker RN, Green NE, Spindler KP. Stress fractures in skeletally immature patients. J Pediatr Orthop 1996; 16:578–584.

19. Lombardo SJ, Retting AC, Lerlan RK. Radiographic abnormalities of the iliac apophysis in adolescent athletes. J Bone Joint Surg 1983; 65A:444–455.

20. Bickerstaff DR, Neal LM, Brennan PO. An investigation into the etiology or irritable hip. Clin Pediatr 1991; 30:6:353–356.

21. Landin LA, Danielsson LG, Wattsgard C. Transient synovitis of the hip. J Bone Joint Surg 1987; 69B:238–242.

22. Illingworth CM. Recurrences of transient synovitis. Arch Dis Child 1983; 58:620–623.

23. Haueisen DC, Weiner SD. The characterization of "transient synovitis of the hip" in children. J Pediatr Orthop 1986; 6:11–17.

24. Sharwood PF. The irritable hip syndrome in children. Acta Orthop Scan 1981; 52:633–638.

25. DeValderrama JAP. The "observation hip" syndrome and its late sequelae. J Bone Joint Surg. 1963; 45B:462–470.

26. Winstrand H. Transient synovitis of the hip in the child. Acta Orthop Scand Suppl. 1986; 57:219.

27. Kallio P, Ryoppy S, Kunnamo I. Transient synovitis and Perthes disease. J Bone Joint Surg 1986; 68B:808–811.

28. DelBeccaro MA, Campoux AN, Bockers T, Mendelman, PM. Septic arthritis versus transient synovitis of the hip: the value of screening laboratory tests. Ann Emerg Med 1992; 21:1418–1422.

29. Kocher MS, Zurakowski D, Kasser JR. Differentiating between septic arthritis and transient synovitis of the hip in children: an evidence based clinical prediction algorithm. J Bone Joint Surg 1999; 81A:1662–1670.

30. Birdi N, Allen U, D' Astous J. Poststreptococcal reactive arthritis mimicking acute septic arthritis: a hospital-based study. J Pediatr Orthop 1995; 15:661–665.

31. Scott, RJ, Christofersen, MR, Robertson WW, Davidson RS, Rankin L, Drummond DS. Acute osteomyelitis in children: a review of 116 cases. J Pediatr Orthop 1990; 10:649–652.

32. Mustafa MM, Saez-Llorens X, McCracken GH, Nelson JD. Acute hematogenous pelvic osteomyelitis in infants and children. Pediatr Infect Dis J 1990; 9:6:416–421.

33. Perlman MH, Patzakis MJ, Jumar PI, Holtom P. The incidence of joint involvement with adjacent osteomyelitis in pediatric patients. Pediatr Orthop 2000; 20:40–43.

34. Viani RM, Bromberg K, Bradley JS. Obturator internus muscle abscess in children: report of seven cases and review. Clin Infect Dis 1999; 28:117–122.

35. Lyon RM, Evanich JD. Culture-negative septic arthritis in children. J Pediatr Orthop 1999; 19:655–659.

36. Ring D, Johnson CE, Wenger DR. Pyogenic infectious spondylitis in children: the convergence of discitis and vertebral osteomyelitis. J Pediatr Orthop 1995; 15:652–660.

37. Hollingworth P. Differential diagnosis and management of hip pain in childhood. Br J Rheumatol 1995; 34:78–82.

38. Jacobsen FS, Sullivan B. Spinal epidural abscesses in children. Orthopaedics 1994; 17:1131–1138.

39. Malhotra R, Singh KD, Bhan S, Dave PK. Primary pyogenic abscess of the psoas muscle. J Bone Joint Surg 1992; 74A:278–284.

40. Rose CD, Fawcett PT, Eppes SC, et al. Pediatric Lyme arthritis: clinical spectrum and outcome. J Pediatr Orthop 1994; 14:238–241.

41. Willis A, Widmann R, Flynn J, et al. Lyme arthritis presenting as acute septic arthritis in children. J Pediatr Orthop 2003; 23:114–118.

42. Jacobs RF, McCarthy RE, Elser JM. Pseudomonas Osteochondritis complicating puncture wounds of the foot in children: a ten-year evaluation. J Infect Dis 1989; 160:657–661.

43. Skaggs DL, Roberts JM, Codsi MJ, et al. Mild gait abnormality and leg discomfort in a child secondary to extradural ganglioneuroma. Am J Orthop 2000; 29:111–114.

44. Tuten HR, Gabos PG, Kumar SJ, Harter GD. The limping child: a manifestation of acute leukemia. J Pediatr Orthop 1998; 18:625–629.

Index